EDITED BY
CARIONA FLAHERTY
& MARION TAYLOR

PRACTICE-BASED LEARNING
for Nursing Associates

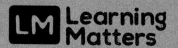

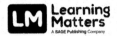

Learning Matters
A SAGE Publishing Company
1 Oliver's Yard
55 City Road
London EC1Y 1SP

SAGE Publications Inc.
2455 Teller Road
Thousand Oaks, California 91320

SAGE Publications India Pvt Ltd
B 1/I 1 Mohan Cooperative Industrial Area
Mathura Road
New Delhi 110 044

SAGE Publications Asia-Pacific Pte Ltd
3 Church Street
#10-04 Samsung Hub
Singapore 049483

Editor: Laura Walmsley
Development editor: Sarah Turpie
Senior project editor: Chris Marke
Project management: River Editorial
Marketing manager: Camille Richmond
Cover design: Wendy Scott
Typeset by: C&M Digitals (P) Ltd, Chennai, India
Printed in the UK

First published 2022

Library of Congress Control Number: 2021942046

British Library Cataloguing in Publication Data

A catalogue record for this book is available from
the British Library.

ISBN 978-1-5297-6309-6
ISBN 978-1-5297-6308-9 (pbk)

At SAGE we take sustainability seriously. Most of our products are printed in the UK using responsibly sourced
papers and boards. When we print overseas we ensure sustainable papers are used as measured by the
PREPS grading system. We undertake an annual audit to monitor our sustainability.

Contents

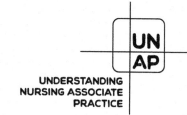

UNDERSTANDING NURSING ASSOCIATE PRACTICE

Supporting you through your nursing associate training & career

UNDERSTANDING NURSING ASSOCIATE PRACTICE is a series uniquely designed for trainee nursing associates.

Each book in the series is:

- Mapped to the NMC standards of proficiency for nursing associates
- Affordable
- Full of practical activities & case studies
- Focused on clearly explaining theory & its application to practice

Other books in the series include:

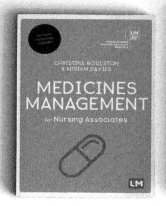
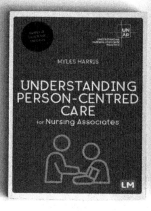
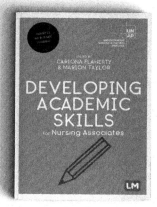

Visit
uk.sagepub.com/UNAP
to see the full collection

About the editors

Cariona Flaherty, RGN, Higher Dip, BSc(Hons), PGCHE, SFHEA, is a senior lecturer in adult nursing and programme leader for Nursing Associates at Middlesex University. Cariona is a specialist trained critical care nurse, who has extensive senior clinical and critical care education experience. In addition to her academic role, Cariona is currently a doctoral student at Middlesex University undertaking research related to critical thinking in undergraduate nurse education.

Marion Taylor, RGN, BEd(Hons), MEd, SFHEA, is an Associate Professor and Director of Programmes at Middlesex University. Marion is an RGN and has a wealth of senior academic experience in leading the development and delivery of nursing and nursing associate programmes. Marion has interest and expertise in supporting students who are also employees, and working in close partnership with employers to ensure students realise their potential.

About the contributors

Mike Bater, RGN, MSc Cancer Nursing, is a senior lecturer in adult nursing and teaches within the Nursing Associate programme at Middlesex University. Mike has a wealth of experience within nursing education and cancer care. Mike has an interest in teaching nursing associates clinical skills and developing their scientific knowledge.

Áine Feeney, RN, BSc(Hons), MA in Practice Education, is a senior lecturer at Middlesex University and teaches across the programme. Áine has extensive experience in ophthalmology and in operating theatres. Practice education is an academic interest of Áine's; she supported learners in practice for several years prior to her academic career.

Pam Hodge, FHEA, is a Lecturer in Practice Learning at Middlesex University. Pam is an RMN who worked in the community across the health and social care divide in practice for many years. Her role focuses on the expansion and quality of nursing student practice learning in non-traditional settings, including social care. Pam's MA thesis focused on how registered nurses in the care home sector engage with educational initiatives to enhance learning in practice.

Adrian Jugdoyl, PG Dip, PGCAP, BSc(Hons), Dip HE (Adult Nursing), Dip HE (Mental Health Nursing), RGN, RMN, NMP, TCH, FHEA, is a senior lecturer and Director of Programmes at Middlesex University. He has extensive experience as an adult nurse, mental health nurse, advanced nurse practitioner and educator and has a particular interest in acute medicine, hepatology and addictions.

Nyamka Marsh, RGN, BSc(Hons), PGCert TPC, is Lead Clinical and Professional Education and Development Nurse for the Nursing Associate programme across North Central London for Primary and Adult Social Care. With a clinical background in practice nursing, she holds the position of borough lead nurse. Nyamka has a special interest in women's health and is enthusiastic about clinical education and the progression and recognition of the nursing team.

Sophie McKay, RSCN, BSc(Hons), Diploma in Tropical Nursing, is an honorary clinical lecturer at Middlesex University and teaches within both the clinical skills and child health teams at the University. She is the paediatric clinical nurse educator at St Mary's Hospital, Imperial College Healthcare Trust. Sophie is a specialist trained paediatric critical care nurse and has a wealth of experience in general paediatrics. Sophie has nursed abroad in Tanzania, Uganda, Mauritius and China.

Sinead Mehigan, RGN, BA(Hons), PGDE, PhD, is head of the Nursing and Midwifery Department at Middlesex University, which delivers programmes for adult, child and veterinary nurses, midwives and nursing associates. With a clinical background in perioperative nursing, she has held positions in clinical practice, clinical education, clinical commissioning, project management and in academia. Academic interests include leadership, anaesthetic and perioperative nursing, preceptorship, workforce development, nursing retention and supporting learners in practice.

Tina Moore is a senior lecturer in adult nursing and is the primary and social care lead within the nursing associate programme. Tina has an abundance of experience within nursing education and continues to work clinically. She also has a special interest in clinical skills and has authored a number of books and articles related to nursing skills and practice.

Aneta Polec, RN, BSc(Hons), PGCert HE (Teaching and Learning), is a lecturer in nursing at Middlesex University. She is a practice and professional modules leader for the Nursing Associate programme across both years. Aneta's experience is in critical care in both practice and education; she also maintains close relationships with medical and surgical wards as a link lecturer. Aneta is currently an MSc student at Middlesex University undertaking research related to experiences of Nursing Associate students in practice.

Esther Reid, RNLD, BN(Hons), MA in Professional Practice, is an Academic Lead at the Institute of Health and Social Care Studies in Guernsey. She also leads on the delivery of the Nursing Associate programme on island; this is offered in partnership with Middlesex University. Prior to her role in academia, she worked in learning disability settings for adults with complex needs and in child and adolescent mental health services for the NHS. She has a keen interest in improving the experiences that people with a learning disability have when they access health and social care services.

Xiaodong Wu, RN, BSc(Hons), MSc in Advanced Nurse Practitioner, NMP, PGCertHE, FHEA, is a part-time lecturer in adult nursing at Middlesex University. He is also currently working in palliative care in the community in North Devon. Previously, he worked at the West London Clinical Comissioning Groups integrated care service, the Marie Curie Hospice and St Joseph's Hospice.

Introduction

This book is designed to support students enrolled on the Nursing Associate (NA) programme, and those supporting them in practice, and in education. However, it is not exclusive to NA students as it includes features that can also support students in undergraduate nurse training or other healthcare programmes who undertake placements in a range of settings.

Who is this book for?

Undertaking placements or experiences in different settings can be a daunting process for NA students who are new to healthcare, and for those who have experience in a different role, but perhaps from one setting. It is a great advantage that NA programmes require and support students to undertake placements in a range of different areas. These allow students to develop their practice, learning and skills development, which will enhance their patient care. However, placements do need to be carefully planned and prepared for, in order to maximise your learning, which this book can help with.

Lecturers and practice education staff who facilitate teaching and learning can use this book. The case studies and activities can be utilised as in-class activities, or pre- or post-sessional work to support the application of new concepts.

About the book

The books starts by exploring the concepts of learning in and from practice, and the process of developing skills in one area of practice that you can transfer to another area: a process known as transferable skills. Following this, the book explores the supportive roles and mechanisms in place for NA students in practice. The remaining chapters then cover some of the most common areas of healthcare practice that provide placement opportunities for students.

It is acknowledged that, as an NA student, you may not attend all of the placement areas addressed in this book during your programme, but you may experience caring for patients with specific needs in other settings. The chapters provide case studies, student tips and activities that enhance your learning and understanding of the different specialties within nursing associate practice.

Book structure

- *Chapter 1, Learning in and from practice,* explores the benefits of different placements; learning in and from placements; how to prepare for placements; and how to look out for transferable skills.
- *Chapter 2, Support in practice,* reviews the support roles and mechanisms in place for NA students in practice, so you are aware of how you will be supported.
- *Chapters 3–10* focus on some of the most common areas of practice that you may have placements in or experience. These chapters can be used as preparatory reading before such a placement. For example, before a placement in social care it would be beneficial to look at Chapter 4 to become familiar with some of the key differences between social care compared to other areas of practice. It is helpful to complete the activities and further reading prior to attending placements so as to have insight into specialist areas of practice. This also will support you in beginning to think about specific learning objectives, for example, what you would like to learn from a specific area, and to consider how this could be useful to you in your own or other areas of practice.

All of the chapters can be used to support you in preparing for placements, but additionally to support your learning when caring for patients in a variety of practice settings. An example of this would be the usefulness of Chapter 6, related to learning disabilities, if you are caring for such a patient in a more general area such as a hospital ward.

Requirements for the NMC Standards of Proficiency for Registered Nursing Associates (NMC, 2018a)

The Nursing and Midwifery Council (NMC) has established standards of proficiency to be met by applicants to different parts of the register, and these are the standards it considers necessary for safe and effective practice. This book is structured to help you understand and meet the proficiencies required for entry to the NMC register as an NA. The relevant proficiencies are presented at the start of each chapter so that you can clearly see which ones the chapter addresses. The proficiencies have been designed to be generic, so they apply to all fields of nursing and all care settings. This is because all NAs must be able to meet the needs of any person they encounter in their practice regardless of their stage of life or health challenges, whether these are mental, physical, cognitive or behavioural.

This book includes the latest standards for 2018 onwards, taken from the Standards of Proficiency for Registered Nursing Associates (NMC, 2018a).

Learning features

Textbooks can be intimidating and learning by reading text is not always easy. However, this series has been designed specifically to help the NA student learn from the books within it. A number of learning features throughout the books will help you to develop your understanding and ability to apply theory to practice, whilst remaining engaging and breaking the text up into manageable chunks. This book contains activities, case studies, student tips, further reading, useful websites and other materials to enable you to participate in your own learning. It cannot provide all the answers – but instead provides a good outline of the most important information and helps you build a framework for your own learning.

It is suggested you read Chapters 1 and 2 as you commence your NA programme and before you begin any module or study sessions related to learning from practice or your placement module, as these chapters provide a useful foundation for this. It is then helpful to read relevant chapters before and during specific related placements to enhance your learning, but also to use as an initial resource or refresher when you are caring for patients with the needs explored, but in different settings, as mentioned above.

We hope that you find this book helpful in supporting you through the practice learning component of your programme of study, and thereafter. Undertaking different placements can provide a number of challenges but it is hoped that this book will support you through this journey and give you the confidence to develop your learning in and from practice.

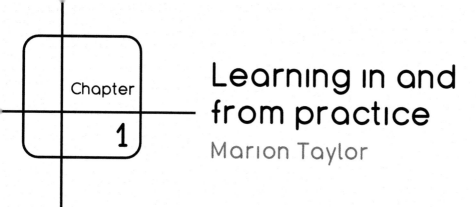

Learning in and from practice

Marion Taylor

NMC STANDARDS OF PROFICIENCY FOR REGISTERED NURSING ASSOCIATES (NMC, 2018A)

This chapter will address the following platforms and proficiencies:

Platform 2: Promoting health and preventing ill health

At the point of registration the Nursing Associate will be able to:

2.1   understand and apply the aims and principles of health promotion, protection and improvement and the prevention of ill health when engaging with people.

2.2   promote preventive health behaviours and provide information to support people to make informed choices to improve their mental, physical and behavioural health and wellbeing.

Platform 3: Provide and monitor care

At the point of registration, the Nursing Associate will be able to:

3.1   demonstrate an understanding of human development from conception to death, to enable delivery of person-centred safe and effective care.

3.2   demonstrate and apply knowledge of body systems and homeostasis, human anatomy and physiology, biology, genomics, pharmacology, social and behavioural sciences when delivering care.

3.3   recognise and apply knowledge of commonly encountered mental, physical, behavioural and cognitive health conditions when delivering care.

3.4   demonstrate the knowledge, communication and relationship management skills required to provide people, families and carers with accurate information that meets their needs before, during and after a range of interventions.

3.6   demonstrate the knowledge, skills and ability to perform a range of nursing procedures and manage devices, to meet people's need for safe, effective and person-centred care.

(Continued)

(Continued)

In order that these proficiencies are achieved, the Nursing and Midwifery Council (NMC) has set Standards for Pre-registration Nursing Associate Programmes (NMC, 2018b). These standards stipulate that programmes must provide opportunities for students to be involved in care delivery across the lifespan and in a variety of settings, and they further specify that this must include children and adults, and patients / service users with mental health conditions and learning disabilities (NMC, 2018b, Section 3).

This context confirms that the Nursing Associate (NA) programme will require all students to undertake a wide range of learning opportunities in different placement areas throughout the programme.

Chapter aims

After reading this chapter you will be able to:

- understand the range of placement areas and why you will be undertaking a range of different placements during your NA programme.
- demonstrate how you can prepare for a placement and maximise your learning during a placement.
- identify the different types of learning in practice and the value of reflection as a tool to support your learning from practice.
- appreciate the role transition required for students with previous healthcare experience.

Introduction

There are a number of clinical placements discussed within this book; as an NA student you may not attend all of the areas addressed in this book during your training. Your placement allocations will be carefully mapped by your university or programme provider to ensure you can achieve the proficiencies mapped out within your Practice Assessment Document (PAD). This chapter will help you as an NA student to understand how you will learn in your practice placements, and how the learning from these placements will enhance your skills in other areas of practice. This can be described as two processes, *learning in practice* and *learning from practice*. These will occur simultaneously in practice, and are explored later in this chapter.

The chapter will firstly explore the range of different placement areas you are likely to experience during your NA programme, and consider the rationale for these different experiences. We will then explore some useful strategies to help you prepare for placements, and to make the most of learning opportunities in areas of practice that are new to you. The concept of learning in practice areas is expanded upon in the later chapters, which relate to some of the more common areas of practice you are likely to undertake. It is helpful to then explore the different ways you will be learning in practice, the principles of transferring learning from one area of practice to another, and the value of reflection as a tool to support this learning.

NA programmes are based in higher education institutions (universities) or employer groups which have been approved by the NMC as meeting the required programme standards (NMC, 2018b). As an NA student you may be undertaking your programme in different ways:

- as an apprentice funded via your employer
- as a seconded student funded by your employer
- as a self-funded student

This affects your employment status and funding situation, but the programme will be the same for all NA students irrespective of the funding route, and all will require you to undertake a range of placements. The placement pattern will ensure a variety of placements, and how these are managed will vary:

- Some programmes have apprentice or employed NA students based in one area of employment who undertake planned placements in different areas during the programme. This is often referred to as a 'hub and spoke' placement model.
- In some programmes apprentice or employed NA students have long experiences in three or four different areas throughout their programme, with no one main employment base.
- Some apprentice or employed NA students work for some days of the week in one area, and have placements in different areas the other days of the week.
- Some NA students who are self-funding will have planned placements in a range of areas, but will not be employees.

These are just some examples of placement patterns; there will be others, but they will all involve the NA student undertaking a range of placements, in order to meet NMC programme requirements (NMC, 2018b). As an NA student you will be supported in practice by a practice supervisor and a practice assessor, as defined by the NMC (2018c; these roles are explored in Chapter 2), as well as a range of other staff.

It is useful to acknowledge that as an NA student you may come across patients with healthcare needs that are not the speciality of the area in which they are being cared for. An example might be a patient who is dying in an area without specific expertise in this, or a patient with mental health care needs in an acute physical care setting. This highlights that the chapters of this book can be useful to you not only in preparation for a specific placement, but also if you are caring for a patient at any point in any setting. Placement areas are challenging to source, with many competing capacity demands from a range of learners. It may be that you gain experience in mental health in a setting caring for patients with dementia, for example, not an acute mental health setting.

It is important to be open-minded to all learning experiences wherever they present you with an opportunity to develop your knowledge and skills in caring for a wide range of patients. As an NA student you will be unlikely to gain specific placements in all of the areas covered within the chapters of this book, but you will undertake a range of placements, and also care for patients with differing needs in more generalised settings.

It is acknowledged that NA students come to the programme from a variety of backgrounds, some with and some without healthcare experience. For those with healthcare experience it is likely that this is as a healthcare assistant (HCA) or similar role, and whilst there can be some advantages to this, there are also challenges. These include being seen differently, as an NA student, possibly in the same area of employment as previous HCA experience, and moving out of your 'comfort zone' where you will have developed expertise. An additional challenge is the transition to being on a programme that has the goal of professional registration as an NMC registrant, with the requirement to meet the NMC Code (NMC, 2018d). These challenges are discussed within this chapter, and the concept of role transition will be explored.

Before we move on to the types of placements and their rationale, it is useful to reflect on your own experience of different areas of placement or employment and the skills you can draw upon from these.

Activity 1.1   Reflection

As you start the NA programme it is helpful to reflect on your previous experience, and how this can now support you with the practice component of your programme. If you have experience in healthcare, make some notes to show the different areas in which you have worked. For example:

- Were you employed as an HCA?
- Was it a short placement as part of an access course, or was it as a Bank or Agency member of staff?

If you don't have healthcare experience make similar notes on your previous employment or college / school experiences. For these experiences identify useful skills that you can transfer into your current programme.

An outline answer is given at the end of the chapter.

Having looked at your previous experiences and how these provide a foundation for your learning, we will now look at the different types of placements you are likely to experience during your programme, and their rationale.

Types of practice areas

NA students will work in many different areas of the country, and in a range of settings such as rural or inner-city locations. Healthcare services in most areas are likely to include some of the following, with local variations:

- primary care settings such as general practice surgeries or health centres
- community nursing services
- community care trusts
- social care settings such as care homes

- mental health services in a range of settings
- learning disability services in a range of settings
- adult acute care services, usually within a Trust
- palliative care settings
- children and young people services in a range of settings

These are explored in other chapters, in which you will see that there are many further services or specialities within each of these services. As mentioned above, you are unlikely to have planned placements in all of these settings, but you may gain insight even through short experiences. An example would be visiting a social care setting as part of a discharge-planning assessment for a patient. This would support your learning around social care and how this differs from an acute healthcare setting.

The different types of placement are extensive, therefore it is helpful to consider in the following activity the healthcare services in your local environment.

Activity 1.2   Evidence-based practice and research

Review the organisation of healthcare services within your location, which can easily be found online. What types of services are there from the above list and in addition to these? If possible review the placement areas that will be included in your programme. If there is an acute Trust, what services or specialities are there within it?

An outline answer is given at the end of the chapter.

Having considered the healthcare settings in your area, it is helpful to now consider why you as an NA student will be having experiences in such different areas. The immediate response to this question could be that it is a programme requirement for all NA programmes, as set out in the NMC Standards for Pre-registration Nursing Associate Programmes (NMC, 2018b) identified at the start of this chapter.

However, we need to explore why the NMC have set this standard, and identified that the NA is a 'generic role', not a field-specific role. To understand this it is helpful to know that registered nurses (RNs) attain their qualification in one of the four fields of nursing – adult, mental health, children and young people and learning disability – and spend the majority of their placements during their programme in a range of areas within this field. These are valuable qualifications, and RNs develop expertise within this field of nursing on registration, but they will have had only limited exposure to the other fields. An example would be an RN Mental Health, who is an expert within their field, but who has had only limited experience of providing physical care skills during their training. They move jobs, remaining in mental health, but in a ward setting in which many patients require physical care, and they need to relearn and develop these skills.

In comparison, the NA role is designed to be generic, not field-specific, thus does not have a field attached to the qualification achieved on programme completion, or the NMC registration. The NA programme ensures you as a student will have experiences in all four fields of nursing, so that you will be able to care for patients in a more holistic way. This is important, as patients or service users and their healthcare needs are not 'neatly packaged' within a field of nursing. For example:

- a patient being cared for by a district nursing team for her leg ulcers who is becoming withdrawn and depressed
- a service user with learning disabilities who needs emergency surgery in an acute setting
- a service user in a mental health setting who develops type 2 diabetes
- a young single mother being cared for within a community mental health service who is worried her child is not developing normally

As these examples show, many patients have multiple and complex needs which cross the boundaries of nursing fields. The chapters in this book relate to different care settings, but as above you will see patients being cared for outside the setting. For example, Chapter 9, on palliative care, will be useful when faced with caring for the dying patient in a different setting, whereas Chapter 9 on mental health can be useful for an accident and emergency experience.

In the following case study we will review if the generic role of the NA and the required placements make sense to you, by exploring if you could explain them to someone else.

Case study: Sampson

Sampson is applying to do his NA programme as an apprentice in the same university and employer as you, an acute Trust, working in a rehabilitation ward. He is keen to do the programme after working as an HCA for 7 years, but he does not understand why he needs to do different placements during his programme. He says he is an expert in his ward, the patients respond to his care well and he always gets good feedback from the team and his manager about his work. He asks you: *Why do I need to do other placements where I won't know anything? I only want to work here when I qualify.*

Activity 1.3   Critical thinking

Make some notes on the key points you would use in your response to Sampson. What potential situations in his ward would benefit from insight and skills gained in other care settings?

An outline answer is given at the end of the chapter.

Now we have discussed the basis for you doing different placements, we will explore how you can make the best of your placements.

Preparing for placements and maximising your learning

We will begin with an activity which will explore how you might feel being presented with a placement allocation.

Activity 1.4   Critical thinking

Imagine you are allocated to a placement next week in an unfamiliar setting. It is unfamiliar in terms of the nursing service and location. What are your initial thoughts and feelings?

Do this by making notes to identify what you need to find out and what types of things you want to learn.

An outline answer is given at the end of the chapter.

Having considered how you might feel when presented with an unfamiliar placement and some initial thoughts on what you need to find out, we will now explore some strategies for addressing this.

These can broadly be grouped in three areas:

- travel and shift times
- nursing service provided
- gaining familiarity with key information

Travel and shift times

You will be provided with some essential information about your allocated placement areas, which will include the exact name of the ward / department / home / GP / service, location, nearest travel links and shift start times. This is all useful, and allows you to start your planning. Use relevant maps or websites to become familiar with the location, and consider this in relation to where you live. Is it a long walk, a bus ride or a more complex journey of tubes and buses involving connections or changes? If a walk is possible, that is always an advantage in terms of the health benefits of exercise and fresh air, but also because the timing is in your control. You can do a practice walk to establish timing, and that is unlikely to alter greatly, allowing you to plan an accurate leaving and arrival time. The shift start time is essential for this, and for most areas this means the time you must be ready in uniform to commence work, often with a handover from the previous shift.

Nursing service provided

Along with the travel and shift information you will be provided with the name of the nursing team. This will take different forms, for example:

- It might be the name of a ward or department if in a hospital base. This should include which Trust the placement is with as some hospital sites have a number of different Trusts on the same geographical site.
- It might be the specific name of a social care setting; for example, Greenlands Lodge.
- It might be the name of a specific service in a mental health organisation; for example, Recovery and Rehabilitation.
- It might be the name of a specific team; for example, District Nursing Team C.

From this you may be able to establish the type of nursing service it provides, for example, Medical Assessment Unit, Cardiac Ward or District Nursing, but other names may not be as obvious. If this is the case you will need to ascertain the type of nursing service provided. You may be able to seek this information from the organisation website, from other students in your group, from your lecturers or by phoning the area. You can also use the National Health Service (NHS) website to search for services local to you: www.nhs.uk/using-the-nhs/nhs-services/ (accessed 4 January 2021).

We will now explore what you can do with this information to further your learning around the speciality of the area.

Student tip 1.1

It's really worthwhile doing a bit of prep before a placement; it only takes a short time but you feel so much better if you do this! For me it was always important to get my travel sorted and my shift times. Having just that basic information made me feel much better, and more in control, especially when going to a completely different area of the city, or to a GP practice, compared to my previous experiences which were all ward-based.

Simone, Year 1 NA student

Gaining familiarity with key information

Look back at your notes from Activity 1.3. They probably include that you need to find out about the type of nursing, as explored above, but then to also learn key terms and concepts related to that area. It can be daunting to go into a new placement area without some understanding of the terminology you are likely to come across, and you are very unlikely to learn if you are feeling nervous and unsure of things because you simply don't understand what is being said. Spending time on this before your placement will be very valuable, and will increase your confidence before you start. Useful resources for this include:

- the relevant chapter within this textbook
- a student pack for the area if available
- patient or service user-facing information, such as relevant national organisations. These provide excellent information, for the members of the public living with the condition and are very good sources of knowledge for students and staff. Relevant ones are included within individual chapters.

Having looked at how to prepare for placements, we will now review your knowledge within the following case study and activity.

Case study: Sophie

I had a terrible start to my first placement. Everything seemed to go wrong; I'm not sure why. I had the information about the placement, and thought I'd try and get there nice and early as I didn't know what time their shifts started. I got to the hospital and couldn't find the ward, asked a few people and eventually was told that I was in the wrong hospital, that the ward I wanted was at another site, although part of the same Trust. So I then had to find a bus to get across to the other site, so rather than being early, I was quite late. The ward were not sure if I was going to arrive or not, as I'd not made contact the week before, which they need new students to do. They said this was shown on the placement information sheet, but I'd only looked at it on my phone so I'd missed that bit. The reason they want you to make contact the week before is to provide some information, and explain the dress code. I realised I was the only one in uniform, so stood out a bit. It was a mental health setting and they do not wear uniforms, so I felt quite uncomfortable. I didn't know it was a mental health area as the Trust has these services as well as acute care services, so that was a bit of a shock!

Activity 1.5   Critical thinking

Having read the case study it is apparent that Sophie did not prepare well for this placement, which put her at a disadvantage. List four things that you think would have made a positive difference to her placement.

An outline answer is given at the end of the chapter.

Having discussed the importance of preparing for your placements, we will now consider maximising your learning during your placement.

Making the most of your placements

Different students can go to the same placement area, even at the same time, and have a very different experience. You may have seen this in your previous employment, or even in school or college. Some students seem to have a positive experience, and others a negative experience, of the same ward, or course or activity. The next activity explores why this might happen.

Activity 1.6   Critical thinking

Make notes on what factors you think influence why some students have a negative experience of a placement, and others a positive one.

You can review your notes as we now discuss some potential factors.

As this activity is based on your own observations there is no outline answer at the end of the chapter.

- How students *commence the placement* is a key factor. If students prepare as suggested in the previous section, they will have a smoother start. They will be on time, not stressed by a late arrival, and will know something of the area and the type of ward or department or service. These students are likely to feel they are able to learn early in the placement, thus maximising their learning.
- How students *communicate and engage* with staff and patients / service users is something that is picked up on fairly quickly after commencement of the placement. Some students do not want to talk with their patients, only to provide the care required, with limited interaction. These students are only gaining some of the potential learning in the area. Talking to patients is hugely important in terms of what you can learn about the impact of a disease or condition on the person's life, and is also enjoyable, thus again maximising both learning and enjoyment of the placement.
- Students' *professionalism and punctuality* are important in terms of how others in the team relate to them as a learner. A student who is always late, on their phone, or asking to change shifts and leave early does not come across as an interested learner, and staff may feel the student does not want to learn, and may not be as keen to teach them.
- Students' *interest in the area* is apparent to their practice assessor, practice supervisor and team members very early in a placement. Some students feel that if the area is one they do not want to work in on qualification there is nothing for them to learn, and some even tell the staff this, which may not engender a willingness for the staff to teach them. Other students have a more open-minded approach, and an attitude of 'wonder what I can learn here?' This means they are not closed to the idea of learning and will enjoy a placement, even if it is one they may not choose to work in when registered.

These examples show that students' preparedness, attitude and mind set contribute to how they experience a placement, and thus explain why some have a positive and some a negative experience of the same ward. However there will be occasions when students have personal challenges or health issues which are impacting on their ability to focus on their learning. They may demonstrate some of the negative traits as above, but this may be because they have personal concerns rather than a lack of interest. It is always adviseable to identify any such challenges to your practice assessor or supervisor so they are aware and can support you appropriately.

Now we have considered some of the components of preparing for your placement and making the most of an experience, we will discuss how you will be learning in practice.

Learning in and from practice

Different ways of learning in practice

Learning in practice is a different way of learning for many students, and differs from learning a theoretical subject. There are many ways of learning in practice. The three explored in this section are:

- working with others to provide care within the proficiencies identified in your PAD
- identifying key learning objectives
- following a patient's journey

Whilst NA practice requires theoretical knowledge which you will gain in university, it is also a practical role. This means you need to develop your competence and confidence in a wide range of care-giving skills which can only be developed by *doing them* in a supported way in practice. Consider when you have learned to drive a car, make a cake or do the ironing, and how you learned this or a similar skill. There may have been some reading and learning on the subject (highway code, recipe book, iron instructions in the examples above), but then you would have engaged with the activity itself, hopefully with some support. NA practice is of course a lot more complex than these examples, as it involves a wide range of skills at any one time, and human interactions with your colleagues, team and patients. However, the principle is the same, in that you cannot learn your NA role without being immersed in practice and begin 'doing it' – undertaking patient care yourself with support. The nature of that support is explored in Chapter 2, but we will now discuss useful processes to facilitate your learning in practice.

Working with others to provide care within the proficiencies identified in your Practice Assessment Document

The NA PAD (PLPLG, 2019) is a document used to both guide and assess your learning in practice. This means it shows what areas of care you will develop proficiency in, and to what level this is required. It also shows the professional values expected of you as an NA student at all times. It is essential to become familiar with this document before your placements, and you will be supported in this. Your practice supervisor, practice assessor and other team members will support your work in practice to ensure you meet the proficiencies possible within each area. If you are familiar with the proficiencies within the PAD you will be able to look out for relevant learning opportunities to complete these. There are 34 proficiencies, and examples of ones you may be able to gain confidence with initially include: providing hygiene care, undertaking patients' observations, collecting specimens, measuring height and weight, supporting patients with eating and drinking. You will initially do these with supervision, or working as a pair with a colleague, and then as you develop competence and confidence, begin to do them independently, with support when needed. This process will be facilitated throughout your programme and can be captured as a learning continuum, as shown in Table 1.1 using the example of undertaking clinical observations.

Table 1.1 Learning in practice continuum

Initial learning	Observation	Undertaking with support	Review	Reflective practice	Developing competence and confidence
Reading and learning related to the skill	Observe the skill being performed by others	Undertake the skill whilst being supported and observed	Review your previous reading and learn to consolidate your knowledge and address any gaps	Undertake the skill independently, seeking advice when needed and reflecting on your practice	Undertake the skill in more complex situations, seeking advice when needed

As you progress through your placements and programme this continuum will be happening for a range of proficiencies at different stages, so for some you might be at the reflective practice level, whilst also learning new skills at the observation stage. Reflective practice is considered in the next section. This continuum is a useful tool to manage your learning, and where possible, to work through the stages. The stages can be fairly quick and seamless and you will soon become comfortable with learning a range of aspects of care giving appropriate to the setting you are in.

It is helpful to review your PAD before each placement and identify the proficiencies that you think are likely to be achieved there, in order to discuss these with your personal assessor at the start of your placement. Some proficiencies cannot be achieved in some placements, but over the course of your programme all will be achieved due to the range of placements you will experience.

Identifying key learning objectives

As well as developing your competence and confidence in your professional values and NA proficiencies, there will be valuable aspects of learning in each placement that are unique to that area. These make each placement different, interesting and enjoyable, and should be welcomed by you as an NA student. It is useful to begin each placement with an idea of what you'd like to achieve in terms of your NA proficiencies, but also specific learning points that relate to the area, which interest you or can inform your future practice. The few examples below are specifically related to the area of care, but these are just examples and each placement area will have many learning opportunities:

- smoking cessation clinic in a GP centre
- planning weekly activities within a care home
- de-escalation techniques within a mental health setting
- planning for patient discharge within a ward setting
- initial assessment by a district nursing team of a patient discharged from hospital
- patient positions used in the operating theatre

The learning opportunities within these different areas are explored in the relevant chapters in this book, so looking at those will provide you with some ideas. The chapters also explore how such learning can be transferable to other areas of practice, thus informing your patient care in your own or other placement areas. The next activity looks at this transferable learning.

Activity 1.7   Work-based learning

Consider the learning opportunities above and identify what other areas of practice this learning is transferable to.

An outline answer is given at the end of the chapter.

There are many other ways of learning in practice, but the final one we will now consider is following a patient's journey. This is a valuable process, although its value as a learning opportunity may not be immediately obvious, so it is worth highlighting.

Following a patient's journey

When working in any area of practice you see one episode or bit of patient care in a whole series of interventions along their healthcare journey. As an NA you will develop considerable expertise within your own area of practice, but will not often have the opportunity to see the other parts of the patient's experience. As a student you do have such opportunities, and it is helpful to take these whenever possible. A local example would be accompanying a patient from a ward to a specialised area such as the operating theatre for endoscopy, remaining and observing the procedure and the patient care provided, and then staying with the patient as they return to the ward, and being involved in their care at this stage. Equally, this can be reversed and a learner from theatre could attend the ward to observe pre- and postoperative care. A further example would be a service user in a mental health setting who is attending a group intervention. These can be managed fairly easily as a learning opportunity by negotiating with your personal assessor and personal supervisor and identifying a suitable patient / service user and date for this. Do look out for similar opportunities as they will always enhance your learning of what the patient has experienced, and also have the benefit of continuity of care for the patient.

A wider experience that allows you to see the patient within a different service can also be useful. Examples include seeing a service user in a community setting from your own hospital setting and vice versa. Again this can be set up with a suitable service user and with negotiation from both teams.

We will now move on to learning from practice by using reflection as a tool to enhance this.

Learning from practice: reflection

Following learning opportunities and shifts in practice it is useful to reflect on your learning, your interactions and your skills development. Reflection is a way of thinking about the event in a structured and managed way to enhance your learning and is explored for NA students by Mehigan (2021, cited in Flaherty and Taylor, 2021).

Using a reflective model allows you to look back on an event, consider it carefully and think about what could be done differently in the future. This can capture positive take-home learning points from situations. For example, I was pleased with how I sat and talked with the patient and encouraged her with her tea; it went well – I must remember that. Learning points may also be negative but informing: That wasn't great. I should not have talked to that service user whilst she was angry and upset. I should have waited until she was calmer. It does not need to be a substantial piece of work or essay, but a reflective piece which you can save in your portfolio, as discussed for NA students by Taylor (2021, cited in Flaherty and Taylor, 2021).

Student tip 1.2

I'd learned about reflection in university and I found it very interesting, and a good way for me to learn, and I found Wright's model the easiest one for me. But it was not always possible to sit and reflect in the middle of a busy shift. In these situations I found it helpful to just take 5 minutes to sit and make a few notes, either on my phone or on paper, and then reflect and write up more fully that evening. I also found it helpful to look back on my reflections to see my learning over a few months – very motivating! This worked for me so it might for you also!

Agnes, Year 2 NA student

Learning from observing in a structured way from role models

A further way of learning from practice worth highlighting is the benefit of learning from positive role models, using some structure to support this; for example, observing a complex or challenging communication interaction between a nurse or NA and a patient or relative. This process is enhanced if the person can discuss it with you beforehand, and give you cues as to what to look out for. You then observe the interaction, and discuss it afterwards. So you can see this has similarities to reflection, but is done together with another person. Learning from role models is a hugely beneficial way of learning skills that are very difficult to learn in other ways. There are many examples of this, including working with an RN or registered NA who says:

- *Join me to talk to this angry relative, and look out for techniques I use to calm her down. We'll discuss your observations afterwards.*
- *Observe this conversation which delivers bad news to a young lady and her husband. We'll chat about it afterwards. Look out for my non-verbal communication especially.*

Having looked at some useful ways of learning from practice, including reflection and observation, we will now consider your transition into the role of being an NA student.

Exploring role transition

Students will have come to the NA programme from a variety of routes. Many will have worked in healthcare as an HCA or in a similar role. If this relates to you it is worth exploring in this section, starting with the next activity.

Activity 1.8   Critical thinking

Write a list of advantages of your previous experience as an HCA.
An outline answer is given at the end of the chapter.

As well as these advantages there are also challenges, and these relate to the transition you are making from an employee in an HCA role into being an NA student. In order to be able to gain all you can from being a student, you need to see yourself differently, and the team you work with need to as well. You may be working with a team you have been in for many years, or a new team. There are some practical things that can support this transition, and will help you develop the mind set of being a student. These include:

- new name badge showing your new role
- new role showing on the off-duty rota, notice board or similar tools
- a different uniform if that is local policy

Your manager will need to be aware of your programme information such as university attendance requirements and placement dates, so do discuss these with them.
It is also important that you take practical steps to support your transition, including:

- ensuring you have your PAD with you at all times
- wearing correct NA student name badge and uniform
- introducing yourself as an NA student (or local title)
- asking questions and having a notebook with you to make notes of things you need to look up later

Student tip 1.3

I'd worked as an HCA for 7 years in my ward, and then became an NA student in the same ward. This was quite weird at first, and I had to make a real effort to see myself as a student, in order to help my colleagues, who I knew really well, to see me as a student as well. I had to be very organised, and asked a lot more questions in order to learn and get my proficiencies signed off in my PAD. I am an apprentice, so still part of the ward team, but everyone now knows I'm a student, and they are keen for me to learn and develop in the role. It took a while, but be patient, and remember you have to make the transition and see yourself as a student before others can.

Maureen, Year 1 NA student

You will gain support with the transition you are making from your university lecturers and education team. It is a process that takes time, and the steps explored in this section will support the process. It is not realistic to simply start a course, have a different badge or uniform and expect to feel like a student. As explored earlier in this chapter, reflection is a useful tool here, with the focus being on what has gone well in supporting your transition, what has hampered this and what could improve in a future situation.

Chapter summary

This chapter has introduced you to how you can learn in practice as an NA student. It has explored why a range of placements are required and useful, and how to prepare for them, using activities to further your understanding. The different ways of learning in practice have been explored, with some advice on maximising your potential to learn. Reflection has been identified as a useful tool to support and develop your learning from practice. Making the transition into being an NA student, especially from an HCA, was explored. Chapter 2 follows on from this and discusses how you will be supported in practice, and subsequent chapters focus on the different areas you are likely to experience in your programme.

Activities: brief outline answers

Activity 1.1 Reflection

Your answer here will identify your experience, so will be individual. For those with healthcare experience, examples could be your time spent in different settings, such as the examples below, with some skills that could be transferred from these experiences:

- Three months on a medical ward as a Bank HCA: skills from this are my patient care skills such as hygiene observations, listening to handovers, working as part of a team.
- Worked in theatres and also included recovery nursing care, and transfers to and from the wards: skills from this are my infection control skills and knowledge, my postoperative care, pain management and moving patients between departments.
- Worked in a community team as part of my access course: this was my first time working with patients and as part of a nursing team, so I learned lots of terminology and gained confidence in talking with patients.

If you haven't worked in healthcare before, you may have gained skills from school or college, for example, studying skills, working in a team, how to research a topic, doing group work with other students.

Activity 1.2 Evidence-based practice and research

Answers to this will vary depending on locality but are likely to include named specifics of:

- local GP surgeries or health centres
- hospital Trusts, and whether these are acute adult or mental health Trusts
- what wards or services can you see on the Trust website?
- district nursing teams: how are they organised?
- what social care settings are there, such as care homes?
- are there learning disability services such as day centres?
- adult acute care services, usually within a Trust
- Are there any hospices or palliative care teams?

Activity 1.3 Critical thinking

You can advise Sampson that although he has a lot of knowledge and skills in his one area of practice, he will need to work in different areas in order to complete all of the proficiencies in his PAD. He also needs to have experience in different settings such as hospitals, community, primary and social care. He needs to ensure he gains experience in each of the four fields of nursing – adult, mental health, children and learning disability. You can also suggest to him that going to different placement areas is enjoyable and interesting, and there is always something to learn from different areas that could impact on your own practice or your own learning and development as an NA.

Activity 1.4 Critical thinking

Your thoughts and feelings will be personal to you, but in terms of what you need to find out your review should include:

- shift times
- travel details
- who to report to
- uniform or dress code requirements
- type of nursing service / care provided
- any key documents to read before the placement

Activity 1.5 Critical thinking

Sophie did not do the following:

- make proper contact with the area in advance of her placement
- find out the exact location
- find out the uniform or dress code
- find out that this was a mental health setting

If she had done these, she would have had a more positive start to the placement and learning experience.

Activity 1.7 Work-based learning

The other areas of practice this learning is transferable to include the following:

- Smoking cessation clinic in a GP centre – this could be useful in any setting to support a patient trying to stop smoking. There will also be skills gained in running a group and providing health promotion to patients that will be useful in many settings.
- Planning weekly activities within a care home – this will develop your organisational skills and skills involved in working with others in a team project.
- De-escalation techniques within a mental health setting – this will allow you to learn skills that can be transferred to other settings where a service user may be angry or agitated, such as in accident and emergency.
- Planning for patient discharge within a ward setting – this will inform you how patients are discharged from hospital, which is useful knowledge when working in a community setting.
- Initial assessment by a district nursing team of a patient discharged from hospital – this is the opposite of the above. It will enhance your knowledge of what information a district nursing team needs when they accept a patient into their care and this can be then used if you are working in a hospital setting preparing patients for discharge.
- Patient positions used in the operating theatre – this provides a useful insight as to aspects of postoperative pain, as some of this relates not to the operation itself, but the position used for surgery, thus can enhance your postoperative care in a surgical ward.

Activity 1.8 Critical thinking

You may have identified a number of advantages, most commonly:

- familiarity with care-giving skills and terminology
- confidence in talking with patients and team members
- knowledge of ward or departmental routines
- previous training such as infection control or basic life support

Annotated further reading

Mehigan, S. (2021) Reflective writing. In: Flaherty, C. and Taylor, M. (eds.) Developing Academic Skills for Nursing Associates. London: Learning Matters, pp. 75–86.

This is a useful chapter with relevant examples of reflective writing for NA students. It explores the value of reflection and models of reflection.

Taylor, M. (2021) Portfolio development. In Flaherty, C. and Taylor, M. (eds.) *Developing Academic Skills for Nursing Associates*. London: Learning Matters, pp. 141–154.

This chapter looks at the value of developing and keeping a portfolio as an NA student and taking this forward into your role as a registered NA. It offers a format for the portfolio, and provides practical tips on commencing this.

Annotated useful websites

This website provides a good overview of the different services within the NHS, and you can also use it to research the services within your local area.

www.nhs.uk/using-the-nhs/nhs-services/

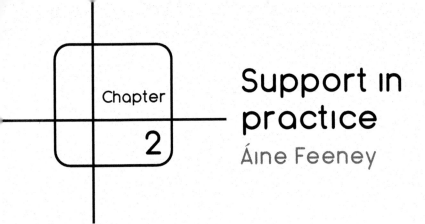

Support in practice

Áine Feeney

NMC STANDARDS OF PROFICIENCY FOR REGISTERED NURSING ASSOCIATES (NMC, 2018A)

This chapter will address the following platforms and proficiencies:

Platform 1: Being an accountable professional

1.11 Understand and act in accordance with the Code: Professional standards of practice and behaviour of nurses, midwives and nursing associates, and fulfil all registration requirements.

1.13 Demonstrate the numeracy, literacy, digital and technological skills required to meet the needs of people in their care to ensure safe and effective practice.

1.14 Demonstrate the ability to keep complete, clear, accurate and timely records.

1.15 Take responsibility for continuous self-reflection, seeking and responding to support and feedback to develop professional skills and knowledge.

1.17 Safely demonstrate evidence-based practice in all skills and procedures stated in Annexes A and B.

Platform 4: Working in teams

4.1 Demonstrate an awareness of the roles, responsibilities and scope of practice of different members of the nursing and interdisciplinary team, and their own role in it.

4.2 Demonstrate an ability to support and motivate other members of the care team and interact confidently with them.

4.7 Support, supervise and act as a role model to Nursing Associate students, healthcare support workers and those new to care roles, review the quality of the care they provide, promoting reflection and providing constructive feedback.

4.8 Contribute to team reflection activities, to promote improvement in practice and services.

Standards for Student Supervision and Assessment (NMC, 2018c)

This chapter focuses on the support the Nursing Associate (NA) student will receive whilst in practice. The Nursing and Midwifery Council (NMC) (2018c) Standards for Student Supervision and Assessment will be used to demonstrate the support available. These standards fall under the following three headings:

- effective practice learning
- supervision of students
- assessment of students and confirmation of proficiency

Chapter aims

After reading through this chapter you will:

- be aware of the people and the resources available to support your learning in practice.
- be guided on how to develop your own learning objectives for different placements.
- be able to develop strategies for looking after and maintaining your own personal health and wellbeing.
- begin to explore resilience.

Introduction

This chapter will explore the different areas of support that are in place and available to you in your practice placements. Chapter 1 has explained the importance of different placements in order for you to meet the requirements of your role. Individual universities or programme teams will arrange placements differently, but your experience in different areas will always meet the NMC (2018c) standards and the support offered will be the same.

There are many people and resources available to you in your NA student role. According to the NMC Code (NMC, 2018d), registered nurses and NAs have a responsibility to support learners in practice. Some will have more specific roles to support your learning as they have undertaken further study to do so in a more recognised capacity. Each of these roles will be described in this chapter, and what you can expect from these individuals is explored.

For every placement you attend you will need to identify learning objectives to be achieved during your placement. These objectives will be personal to you and will be based on your learning needs but also on the specialty of the area. This chapter will give you guidance on how to prepare these learning objectives.

As an NA student working towards registration you also need to take personal responsibility for the maintenance of your own personal health and wellbeing. You are a student on a healthcare programme and therefore there is an expectation that you 'practise what you preach' with regard to health and wellbeing. The NMC (2018d) require this of all registrants and students, and this will be explored in this chapter.

Resilience is an important part of being a healthcare professional and this concept will be introduced in this chapter with some suggestions on how you can build and achieve resilience.

Support in practice: the people and resources

There are three main roles identified to support students in practice. These are:

- practice supervisor (PS)
- practice assessor (PA)
- academic assessor (AA)

Each of these roles is discussed here in addition to other staff available to support you.

Practice supervisor

On arrival at your placement you will be allocated a PS. This will be a registered member of the healthcare team. As an NA student you will be supervised while learning in practice. This will generally be by a registered NA or a registered nurse (RN); however in some placement areas you may find that there are no registered NAs (RNA) or RNs, and you will be allocated a different registered healthcare professional as your PS. Can you think of who else in your work area is a healthcare professional with registration to a professional body? This could be a doctor, podiatrist, dietician, operating department practitioner, radiologist or many others. Your PS needs to know about the programme you are studying on in order to support you appropriately.

The role of a PS is to be a role model for you in practice by demonstrating safe and effective practice. Your PS will support your learning within the limits of their own scope of practice. You should expect to be supported, supervised and given feedback on your progress. All of this support and feedback is essential for your progress in achieving confidence, competence, proficiencies and skills. In turn, your PS must keep up to date and remain current in their practice while also receiving support for facilitating your learning. Your PS is supporting you as part of their role; the care of the patient is paramount and your understanding of their role in supporting you is essential for the delivery of safe and effective care. In addition to supporting you in practice your PS will contribute to your Practice Assessment Document (PAD) and record relevant information within that. They will also liaise with your PA and AA to share details of your performance related to both practice and professional conduct. For example, at the midway and final assessments in your PAD your PA will discuss and collate all relevant information on your conduct and competence to date on your placement.

There is no set guidance outlined by the NMC for how much time you should be spending with your PS. You may work with them on every shift or less than this.

During your placement there will be many staff you can work with and you must ensure that you have an appropriate registered practitioner to report to if you have any concerns during a shift/placement. Other registered staff can support you and they will also be approached for feedback on your performance, contributing to your overall placement assessment.

Practice assessor

You will be assigned a PA in the placement areas that you are allocated to. This PA must be an RN or an RNA. This PA may cover one or a series of placements; this will depend on the arrangements that your university and the placement areas have decided. Your PA will complete the assessment components of your PAD with you and collate information from your PS, other staff and health professionals that you have been working with and learning from. It is the role of the PA to assess your performance in practice to achieve the proficiencies and programme outcomes for practice learning. You may not work directly with your PA each day; however there will be sufficient opportunities for your PA to observe your practice so that they can inform the decisions made for your assessment and your progression on your programme.

It is important for you to know that your PS and your PA cannot be the same individual. This requirement from the NMC (2018c) reduces any bias that one individual acting as both your supervisor and assessor may have with regard to your practice and your learning during a set period of time.

Academic Assessor

As part of the NMC Standards for Student Supervision and Assessment (2018c), each student will have an AA for each part of their programme. This AA will be an RN from your university. The AA will work closely with your PA by communication and collaboration at relevant points in the programme related to student progression. Each university may assign the AA in different ways. You may find that your AA is your personal tutor, your link lecturer and/or your Apprenticeship Tripartite reviewer. This individual is also an essential resource for you with regard to your learning and can be approached by you for guidance and pastoral support throughout your studies.

Manager

The manager in your placement will also be a valuable person supporting your learning. They may not be your PS or PA but they will facilitate your learning in many ways. There will be many learning opportunities on your placement and the manager will be aware of all of the personnel and the patients with whom you will be working and can help to identify specific learning opportunities for you. The manager in the area will also be available to support your PS and PA in their roles. Achieving your protected learning time will be one of your priorities and the manager will be paramount in understanding and supporting its occurrence.

Practice or clinical educator (or similar title)

The majority of workplaces and placement areas that you will be attending will have a member of the healthcare team who has responsibility for the NA students in their Trust or workplace. This individual may be part of a larger clinical education team depending on the workplace. For example, a hospital will usually have a nursing education team; in contrast, in a GP practice you may find that there is no such team but you will have the name of the professional responsible for your placement. The practice educator is another individual you can approach for support during your placement. The clinical education teams work closely with your university and will help to escalate any concerns related to your learning or the practice placement area.

Other nursing staff will be available to support you during your placements. For the registered nursing team the NMC (2018c) deem that students and learning must be supported in practice. As mentioned previously, patient care is always the priority; however, all RNs and RNAs and in fact students should be available to support other students and learners in their practice area. In a successful learning environment there are many staff willing to help and support you in your learning. Healthcare support workers and other technical staff are also available to facilitate your learning and are vital members of the team from whom you can learn and develop skills related to your placement.

Multidisciplinary team (MDT)

Spending some of your protected learning time with specialist nurses and other members of the multiprofessional team is an ideal way to increase your learning opportunities and you can then use these experiences to complete your reflections. These experiences can be recorded in your PAD and comments included by the healthcare professional will help to influence and consolidate your learning. Each of the chapters in this book refers to the MDT and the learning you can achieve with them in different placement areas.

Case study: Zoe

Zoe is a student NA in Part 1 of her programme. She is on week 3 of a 6-week placement and she is due to complete her midway assessment with her PA Michael at the end of this week. Zoe was not aware that her PS Ruta would be on annual leave for this and the following week. Zoe is not worried or concerned about who will work with her over these weeks as the nursing team are always very supportive, but she is unsure who will be her PS instead of Ruta and who will complete her PAD midway assessment. Zoe rarely ever works with or sees her PA and she is not sure what to do with regard to getting her PAD completed in a timely manner.

Michael is aware that Ruta is away on leave and he has already spoken with her and collated her feedback and comments on Zoe's performance on her placement to date. Ruta had already emailed Zoe the date and time of her midway assessment at the time of her induction and primary meeting.

Activity 2.1   Communication

Read the above case study and consider the following questions:

1. Who can Zoe contact to inform them of her concerns?
2. How will Zoe know who she can work with in Ruta's absence? Who can she report to?
3. Where can Zoe seek further support in her workplace to assist her with her concerns?
4. Does Zoe need to contact her university to inform them of this episode?

An outline answer is given at the end of the chapter.

Developing learning objectives for your placement

As you study academic modules at university you will be familiar with the concept of learning outcomes. Your modules will have specific learning outcomes that you need to achieve through study, attending lectures, linking theory to practice and completing an assessment. For practice you also need to meet learning objectives; these objectives will be set by you and will reflect your stage in your programme, your previous learning and the learning available in the practice area that you will be attending. These different placement areas are covered in subsequent chapters; however it is important that before commencing a placement you review your learning to date, what you need to achieve and whether you can meet this learning objective on your current placement.

For each part of your programme you will have a PAD (PLPLG, 2019). This document forms part of your overall assessment and is essential for your progression. In this document you will record your learning in practice and it is where your PS and PA will document your meetings, assessments and proficiencies. There are a variety of staff who can also contribute to your PAD, such as specialist nurses and other healthcare professionals. The PAD will be submitted through university processes and it will contribute to your overall learning. Completion and submission of your PAD will be essential for you to complete your programme.

Prior to attending your placement you need to identify what you think you are going to learn in and from this experience. It is important that you familiarise yourself with what proficiencies in your PAD you still need to accomplish during this placement. As a student with responsibility for your own learning it is important that you have an overarching knowledge of what you need to complete your PAD. Remember that what you learn in each placement is never learned in isolation. All learning is built on and all transferable skills built upon will add to your overall experience. In Chapter 1 you have explored what you need to do prior to placement so you are prepared for your first day.

Knowing the specialty of the practice area and having identified what skill you have to achieve in this placement are all part of your preparation. You will be meeting with your PA and PS early in your placement to complete your initial meeting. As part of this meeting you will be required to set learning objectives during your placement. These objectives may be influenced by your PS based on the specialty of the area and their knowledge of what is available for you to learn in this placement. For example, if you are going to an ophthalmic unit you will learn about patients with eye conditions and the care of these patients. If you have an outstanding skill to learn about blood transfusions it is highly unlikely that you can complete that skill in this unit.

Some units may have a list of learning objectives that they use for all learners and on meeting your supervisor you can discuss any outstanding skills that you need to achieve. You should also use the feedback provided to you in your previous placements to influence your plans. Your PS will also want to read through your PAD to see if there are previous action plans or recommendations and comments from your previous PA that can influence your learning objectives for this current placement.

Student tip 2.1

Before starting your placement it's a good idea to review the comments and feedback from your PS and PA in your previous placement. If there are comments relating to something to improve on, it's good to focus on this in your next placement. For example, after my first placement I was told that my verbal communication was improving but more confidence was needed when speaking with the multiprofessional team. I thought about ways to improve this in my next placement. One thing I did was to aim to build my confidence during patient handover, so I did as many of these as possible and it really helped! This demonstrated to my PS and PA that I had learned from previous feedback and also showed that I am proactive in my practice learning.

Toni, NA student

Each placement you attend will have many different experiences for you to learn from. Although it is important to achieve the skills identified in your PAD there may be specific areas where there are different skills for you to learn that are not in your PAD. Taking advantage of these learning opportunities will enhance your overall learning on this programme. Take each placement as a separate learning opportunity and avail yourself of all the resources on offer to you. Your skills need to be completed in your PAD but the list of opportunities, learning outcomes and skills is endless. You must only practise within your scope of practice as an NA student; however exposure to the many learning objectives and skills available will depend on your initiative and willingness to learn. Being proactive in your approach to each placement and what learning you will achieve will be influential to your success.

The chapters in this book focus on different placement areas and the types of learning you can achieve in them, which widens your knowledge and also transfers to your practice in other areas, as explored in Chapter 1.

Personal health and wellbeing

According to the NMC Code (2018d), you have a responsibility to maintain your health at a level where you can carry out your professional role. It is important that as a healthcare professional you can identify when your health and wellbeing are compromised. All workplaces will have policies and procedures to follow regarding sick leave and you should be familiar with these. When you are unwell you need to take the appropriate steps to get well. If you are unwell you cannot be expected to continue to perform at the expected level of your competence and therefore taking time off may be essential.

Throughout your programme you will learn about health promotion and public health in addition to social determinants and inequalities of health. You need to consider your own personal health in relation to each of these topics and make all efforts to improve and maintain your own good health and wellbeing as you will be offering this advice to others. Consider yourself working in an outpatient department in a respiratory clinic: if the NA providing health promotion information on smoking cessation has just been outside for a cigarette and has the odour of smoke on their breath and their uniform, how do you think this will influence the patient? Smoking is only one example; there are many more that you can imagine to fit this situation. Being a role model to peers and colleagues is an essential part of your role. As healthcare professionals we need to consider how our health and health behaviours can be interpreted by patients, families and colleagues. Keeping healthy through diet and exercise are of great benefit to you in your busy life; studying and working can be a challenge and looking after your own physical and mental health is a strength that should be promoted by those working in healthcare.

From reading this chapter you have seen that there are many professionals related to your support in practice. It is also worth remembering that you can contact your personal tutor at the university if you feel that you require more individual support regarding your health and wellbeing. Attending tutorials and meetings with your tutor is an important way of facilitating pastoral support, and contacting your personal tutor at times of difficulty may help your overall performance.

Introduction to resilience

Having a level of resilience is seen as useful when working in healthcare. So what is resilience and how do you develop it? When you demonstrate resilience it shows that you can 'bounce back' from an experience; you can 'take things in your stride'. Resilience can be seen as an optimistic view on life, with the ability to experience personal change allowing the person to keep going and outlive the negative experience (McGee, 2006). It does not mean that you have to have negative experiences in order to be resilient. You can learn to be resilient. As a student NA you have already had to accept changes to your work, your study and your personal life. This may have been more of a challenge to others than to you due to different personal circumstances, but how have you managed these changes? By adapting to changes as you commence the NA programme you are demonstrating resilience. Other changes such as attending different placement settings, writing academic assessments and giving verbal presentations are all challenges that you have faced and will continue to face on your educational and professional journey. Everyone experiences these challenges and we all manage them differently. It is true that some students will adapt to these changes sooner than others but you will all face similar challenges in your studies and in your professional career. There are many tools that can be used to assist you in boosting your resilience, including reflection and becoming more self-aware.

The skills for reflection are explored by Mehigan (2021) and taught to you in university and developed further through your written reflections and through many submitted assessments.

Becoming more self-aware is a skill for life that you need to embrace to help you develop into the healthcare professional that you want to become. Mindfulness is a current topic in the public domain and focusing on your own mental health is now seen as a necessity to be considered alongside physical health. This type of learning can only be completed by you as it is to improve and enhance your health and wellbeing. We will now explore these ideas in an activity.

Case study: Chidi

An action plan has been raised at a student NA's midway assessment; she is worried and concerned. Please work through the following activity using a reflective model.

Chidi is a Year 2 NA student on her second 6-week placement. She has been late to placement on several occasions in her first few weeks. Her PS has spoken to her about her poor punctuality and Chidi has promised to do her best to improve. In addition to being late for the start of shifts, Chidi has been returning back from her breaks 5–10 minutes late. Following the discussion with her PS early in her placement, Chidi has not improved her time management. As a result her PS and PA have agreed to implement an action plan in Chidi's PAD on time management and punctuality. At the time of the midway assessment this is raised and Chidi is very upset that being late a couple of times has resulted in an official action plan in her PAD.

Activity 2.2   Reflection

Imagine that you are Chidi, you are struggling with child care for your 3-year-old twins and you have never had a negative action plan before. You are really worried about this and how it will affect your placement and your overall programme. Using a reflective model of your choice, answer the following questions:

- What steps can Chidi take to resolve this situation?
- What can help her to improve her time keeping?
- Who is available to Chidi to help her meet the action plan?
- When will she need to demonstrate an improvement by?
- How would you manage this situation if it were to happen to you?
- What have you learned about how resilience informs this situation?

An outline answer is given at the end of the chapter.

From completing this activity you will have identified numerous ways that you can improve your communication and your relationships with your PS and PA and have demonstrated how reflection can assist you with improving your self-awareness. Learning from personal challenges helps to build resilience and enhance your further learning.

Following this activity we will now summarise the learning from this chapter.

Chapter summary

In this chapter we have identified a number of important topics related to the support that you will have in practice and some strategies to assist you with achieving an enjoyable and informative practice placement while learning and achieving your proficiencies. You now know who is available to support you in your learning in your practice placements. There has been exploration through the activities included to promote your developing confidence through communication, reflection and resilience.

Activities: brief outline answers

Activity 2.1 Communication

1. Who can Zoe contact to inform them of her concerns?

    There are a number of people who Zoe can contact. Contacting her PA (Michael) will help her to identify if he is available for her midway assessment. At this point Michael reminds Zoe that they have an appointment for this review and he suggests that she revisit her emails to view the details. If Zoe is unable to contact Michael, she could contact the ward manager to inform them that she is going to be without a supervisor for the next 2 weeks. The practice education team would also be a source of support if Zoe is unable to resolve this with her manager or her PA.

2. How will Zoe know who she can work with in Ruta's absence? Who can she report to?

    We already know that the staff on the ward are very supportive, so Zoe will have other staff to work with. It is important that Zoe informs the team leaders that her PS is away so that she is adequately supported in her role during this assessment period.

3. Where can Zoe seek further support in her workplace to assist her with her concerns?

    This has been covered in the previous answers.

4. Does Zoe need to contact her university to inform them of this episode?

   It is not necessary on this occasion for Zoe to inform the university. This episode can be resolved locally. However it is important to add that if this situation were to recur it would be important to raise it with the practice education team, who could then support Zoe's concerns and include the university to help resolve the situation.

Activity 2.2 Reflection

This answer uses the Driscoll (1994) model of reflection to answer the questions in the activity.

What? I've been really struggling with child care for the twins as my partner is currently working away from home and it is so difficult to get ready for my early shifts and get the twins ready. I've been late to placement on about three occasions and have apologised each time. Now I'm being told that this is not acceptable and that there will be an official action plan in my PAD. I am so worried about this as in normal circumstances I am always on time and I don't want to fail this placement as I have so much to do at the moment. I know my PS has mentioned I was late but I didn't think it could be this serious.

So what? In the midway assessment I told my PS and PA that I was struggling with child care and I was finding it difficult to be on time. They could tell how upset I was due to my tears in the meeting. They mentioned that I should have told them earlier about the situation as they could potentially have helped me by changing my shift pattern to accommodate my child care. They also told me that we could talk to the practice education team and the university to see what options were available to support me at this time. Overall the message that I took from this meeting was that I should have communicated the difficulties I was having earlier to my PS. I accept that I was late back from my breaks but often this was due to phone calls regarding my child minder.

Now what? I have agreed that I will improve my punctuality for the remainder of my placement as I do not want to fail on these grounds. I have planned for my family to help me more while my partner is away for the next 2 weeks, so that I can focus on my time keeping for the placement. I will plan to complete my breaks and return to practice on time by arranging specific times to speak with my child minder, when possible. According to the action plan I have up to 3 weeks to improve my time keeping and punctuality. I now also know that if I am struggling with anything in my work or personal life that affects my study and my placements, I need to speak to someone about this. The PS is a good person to start with and if they cannot help me they can assist me in finding out who I do need to contact.

Annotated further reading

Rowe, G. (2020) Introduction to mental health and wellbeing writing. In Rowe, G., Counihan, C., Eillis, S., Gee, D., Graham, K., Henderson, M., Barnes, J. and Carter-Bennett, J. (eds.) *The Handbook for Nursing Associates and Assistant Practitioners*, 2nd ed. London: SAGE

This chapter explores resilience in healthcare and suggests ways to help improve your happiness.

Feeney, Á., and Everett, S. (2019) *Understanding Supervision and Assessment in Nursing*. London: SAGE.

Even though this book is aimed at the RN and the RNA with regard to supervision and assessment, you may find it helpful to understand the requirements for the staff supporting you in practice.

Annotated useful websites

This website provides guidance to nurses and NAs on the learning resources available to support student nurses and student NAs in practice.

https://plplg.uk/e-learning-resources/

This NHS website provides an introduction to mindfulness that you may find helpful.

www.nhs.uk/conditions/stress-anxiety-depression/mindfulness/

This website offers ways to become more mindful.
www.mindful.org/

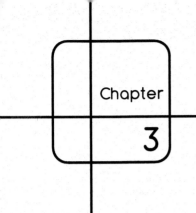

Primary care settings

Tina Moore and Nyamka Marsh

NMC STANDARDS OF PROFICIENCY FOR REGISTERED NURSING ASSOCIATES (NMC, 2018A)

Platform 2: Promoting health and preventing ill health

At the point of registration, the nursing associate will be able to:

2.1 understand and apply the aims and principles of health promotion, protection and improvement and the prevention of ill health when engaging with people.

2.2 promote preventive health behaviours and provide information to support people to make informed choices to improve their mental, physical and behavioural health and wellbeing.

2.7 explain why health screening is important and identify those who are eligible for screening.

Platform 3: Provide and monitor care

At the point of registration, the nursing associate will be able to:

3.5 work in partnership with people, to encourage shared decision making, in order to support individuals, their families and carers to manage their own care when appropriate.

3.7 demonstrate and apply an understanding of how and when to escalate to the appropriate professional for expert help and advice.

3.11 demonstrate the ability to recognise when a person's condition has improved or deteriorated by undertaking health monitoring. Interpret, promptly respond, share findings, and escalate as needed.

Platform 6: Contributing to integrated care

At the point of registration, the nursing associate will be able to:

6.1 understand the roles of the different providers of health and care. Demonstrate the ability to work collaboratively and in partnership with professionals from different agencies in interdisciplinary teams.

6.4 understand the principles and processes involved in supporting people and families with a range of care needs to maintain optimal independence and avoid unnecessary interventions and disruptions to their lives.

Chapter aims

After reading this chapter you will be able to:

- identify the range of primary care services.
- demonstrate knowledge and understanding of the procedures involved in performing NHS Health Checks.
- identify key issues in relation to patient confidentiality and informed consent.
- explain your role as a Nursing Associate (NA) student in the management of recalling patients and escalating concerns.
- identify and use a range of effective communication skills in the management of patient care.

Introduction

This chapter will firstly explore what types of services are included in the umbrella term primary care, which you may have a placement experience in as an NA student. The learning opportunities in primary care settings will then be explored. There are many learning opportunities within this particular area of practice, and a discussion of them all is beyond the remit of this chapter. Therefore, we will concentrate on health promotion and illness prevention, which are pivotal within primary care. The concept of self-management is key to health promotion and will also be discussed, giving consideration as to how these are useful in a range of other settings you may experience. This will include using patient-centred care, health checks and reviews within a multidisciplinary team (MDT). For clarity, within some community settings the term 'service user' or 'patient' may be used. For the purpose of consistency the term 'patient' will be used within this chapter.

The range of primary care provision

Primary care includes services provided by general practice, community-based facilities (e.g. district nursing), school nurses, health visitors, dentistry, occupational therapy and pharmacy. All these services work together to provide an integrated healthcare service for patients.

Primary care networks build on existing primary care services and enable greater provision of better integration of health and social care that is proactive, personalised and coordinated and therefore promotes a shift from providing appointments (reactive) to becoming more proactive and adopting a preventive stance when caring for people within the community.

In general practice, the nurse's role is commonly regarded as complementary to that of the general practitioner (GP), extending activities of general practice through nurse-led services, undertaking an ever wider range of roles and with experienced nurses assuming more of the traditional workload of GPs. Many of these roles are also now being devolved to the NA. There is considerable variation in the tasks undertaken by primary care nurses and their level of responsibility. They are often viewed as a true 'partner in care' and a complementary professional asset in a GP practice.

There are many facets to the role of the primary care nurse or NA. For example:

- clinical activities (Doppler assessment, compression bandaging, wound management, medicines management, ear irrigation)
- assessing and monitoring a patient's health status
- organisational – recall of patients, follow-up of appointments, coordination of patient care
- coordination of care – ensuring patients have the correct service, communicating between different health disciplines and organisations and between patients and health services
- treatment and care of sick individuals
- rehabilitation and disability care
- palliative care
- rapid response (acute care, particularly for those who do not want to be hospitalised or to prevent hospitalisation)
- vaccinations and immunisations (including childhood, travel vaccines, flu vaccines)
- women's health clinics (including cervical screening)
- men's health clinics
- home visits
- chronic illness management
- wound care, Doppler assessment, compression bandaging
- health screening, illness prevention and health promotion
- drug and alcohol treatment and support
- some practice nurses treat minor injuries and minor operations done under local anaesthetic
- running smoking cessation clinics

The role allows nurses / NAs to develop long-term relationships with individuals and families, managing their conditions and improving their physical and mental health and wellbeing. However this is only possible when sufficient time can be invested to support patients in developing effective self-management and preventive measures.

As an NA student working in primary care, you will be expected to participate in a large number of the activities mentioned above. Activity 3.1 explores your current understanding of primary care.

Activity 3.1   Reflection

The NA programme offers a variety of experiences in terms of both theory and practice (placements), including primary care. If you have been allocated to a primary care setting, think of the key learning points for you. Write these down in a spider diagram. Also think about how this learning differed from your normal workplace. If you have not yet been allocated to a primary care setting, what do you expect to learn? Again, write down your answers.

As this activity is based on your own reflection there is no outline answer at the end of the chapter.

The multidisciplinary team within primary care

Working in healthcare requires you to be aware of all other local services available in order to provide patients with a wide breadth of opportunities.

An MDT is a diverse group of professionals who work together to deliver person-centred and coordinated care for patients. The role of the primary care nurse or NA is clarified at the beginning of this chapter, but the list is not exhaustive. Information about various professionals you may find in the MDT is provided below. You will need to keep up to date with local services and the ways to refer as information is constantly changing. Do take every opportunity to work with them in order to gain more insight into their roles.

MTD roles may include the following:

- *GPs* are normally the first point of contact, caring for patients in the community or in their own homes. GPs care for patients with complex care needs (physical, psychological and social).
- *Pharmacists* provide medicines management, preparing and dispensing prescription and non-prescription medicines.
- *Occupational therapists* are involved in the rehabilitation of people who have developed a disability (caused by either physical or psychological illness, the ageing process or accident). Like the pharmacist they manage patients of all ages.
- *District nurses* are practitioners who work in the community visiting people in their own homes or in residential care.
- *Health visitors* (specialist community public health nurses) are responsible for supporting families with children under 5 years of age.
- *School nurses* (specialist community public health nurses) work with schoolchildren providing services such as development screening, immunisation screening and personal, social and health education (including sex education).
- *Community children's nurses* provide care for children who are sick within their own homes.

- *Community mental health nurses* manage people with long-term mental health conditions within the community (adults, children, drug / alcohol addiction).
- *Learning disability nurses* provide specialist healthcare for people with a range of learning disabilities.
- *Physiotherapists* help to restore and maximise movement and function through tailored exercise and physical activity advice.
- *Speech and language therapists (SaLT)* work with people who have speech, language and communication difficulties as well as eating and swallowing problems.

Patient-centred care

As with carrying out procedures, when referring patients to other professionals you must ensure you have gained the patient's consent. You must make sure that the patient understands to whom they are being referred and why, as well as the time frame and next steps (e.g. telephone, video or in-person consultation). All healthcare workers/ professionals are bound by laws and regulations covering many aspects, particularly sharing of information, and should also be aware of local information governance rules and General Data Protection Regulation (GDPR) (2018).

Patient-centred care is paramount to assisting patients with achieving good health outcomes. Below is a helpful tool known as the four As (Public Health England, 2015), which will enable you to structure questions to allow patients to participate in coordinating their own care. There are are also useful tools to enhance the outcomes of NHS Health Check with tips on communication and identifying risk; for example, cognitive assessment tools and alcohol use screening tests.

Four As

1. *Ask* the client about their lifestyle (listen carefully); ask permission to have the conversation.
2. *Advise* using a person-centred approach:
   - 'What concerns you about ...?'
   - 'What do you know about ...?'
   - 'How do you think you would benefit from making a change?'
   - 'What could you do?'
   - 'Where do you think you'll be in a year's time/3 years' time if you don't make a change?'
3. *Assess*: does the client want to make a change?
   - 'Would you like support?'
4. *Assist*: signpost to an appropriate service.

(Public Health England, 2015)

Recalling patients

Recalling a patient is an essential part of the healthcare system, indicating that they are required to attend a follow-up appointment for a number of reasons. Recalls may be routine, like bowel screening or annual reviews, or they may be ad hoc following tests. Whether someone requires a recall appointment depends on a patient's medical history, results and any new information obtained.

There are limited placement opportunities for students, particularly within a GP practice setting. The following case studies are designed to reflect common situations within this practice area and can be used as a resource to aid your learning.

Learning from NHS Health Checks

Purpose of NHS Health Checks

There is no doubt that nurses and NAs play an important role in promoting public health, focusing on disease prevention and behavioural change. Within primary care settings much of this is delivered by NAs and healthcare assistants. This includes health checks, consultation, follow-up treatment, delivery of health promotion, patient education and a strong focus on illness prevention.

Delivery is through an individualised approach that incorporates a behaviour-changing perspective. Overall goals are to prevent disease, reduce symptoms and increase the cost-effectiveness and efficiency of services as well as enhance patients' experiences of health-care services.

Within primary care routine health checks are key in helping to decrease the risk of stroke, heart disease, type 2 diabetes and kidney problems. In addition the tests also help to identify certain types of dementia. Routine health checks occur on a 5-yearly basis.

The evidence of success for this type of approach is undeniable. Taken together, those health conditions identified by the NHS Health Check are the largest cause of preventable deaths in the UK, affecting around seven million people (NHS, 2019a). In fact, in its first 5 years since its implementation, the NHS Health Check is estimated to have prevented 2,500 heart attacks or strokes, as a result of people receiving treatment after their Health Check (NHS, 2019a).

The latest research suggests that:

- for every 30–40 people having an NHS Health Check, one person is diagnosed with hypertension
- for every 80–200 people having a Health Check, one person is diagnosed with type 2 diabetes
- for every 6–10 people having an NHS Health Check, one person is identified as being at high risk of cardiovascular disease

(NHS, 2019a)

The NHS Health Check is offered to everyone aged 40–74 to prevent premature death from:

- heart disease
- stroke
- kidney disease
- diabetes

(NHS, 2019a)

This is achieved by monitoring for warning signs indicating that a patient's level of risk of these health conditions is higher than average. Once a patient has been identified as being at risk of developing co-morbidities (or has already developed them), lifestyle advice can be given, adjusted to individual needs. This is coupled with possible medical treatment in order to reduce the risks.

It is important to note that some warning signs of cardiovascular disease, such as hypertension and hypercholesterolaemia (high cholesterol) are "silent", which means they have no symptoms. So, individuals can feel well even though their risk is raised or indeed high.

As part of your NA programme, you will be introduced to concepts of health promotion that you can apply within your own workplace. We will now look at an example of a lack of health awareness in the case study on Mr Brown.

Case study: Kenneth

During your clinic you receive a phone call from reception letting you know they have just booked a patient into your next empty appointment slot for an NHS Health Check.

The patient is Kenneth, a 74-year-old man. After discussion with the patient you discover that he has no concerns. He states that he is only there because he responded to a request to attend the practice for a routine health check. This will be his first ever health check. He lives with his wife and they have five children, all living at home.

The results of his health check are as follows:

- Height: 5 foot 10 inches (1.78 metres)
- Weight: 14 stones 11 lb (89.6 kg)
- Body mass index (BMI): 29.7
- Blood pressure: 110/69 mmHg
- Waist circumference: 39.5 inches (100.3 cm)
- Smoking status: non-smoker
- Alcohol: 8 units per week
- Past medical history: none
- Family history: no family history of heart disease, mother type 2 diabetic
- Employment: used to work as a concierge but is now retired
- Activity level: he manages to undertake 30–60 minutes of light exercise weekly
- Diet: eats more than five fruit and vegetables a day

Activity 3.2   Critical thinking

- After reading Kenneth's results do you have any concerns? If so, what are they?
- Would you carry out or request any further investigations? If so, which ones?
- What advice would you offer Kenneth?

- Do you think any part of Kenneth's care should be escalated? If so, in what areas and who would you raise your concerns to?
- Can you name any other services you may refer Kenneth to?

An outline answer is given at the end of the chapter.

Learning from reviews

Conducting an asthma review

The UK has one of the worst asthma death rates in Europe, with deaths having increased by more than 33% in the last decade (Asthma UK, 2019). It is known within primary care that self-management reduces emergency use of healthcare resources, including emergency department visits, hospital admissions and unscheduled consultations, and improves markers of asthma control, including reduced symptoms and days off work, and, importantly, improves quality of life. This supports the requirement for continued asthma reviews, self-management education and follow-up appointments.

Asthma is a long-term condition/chronic disease that is characterised by inflammation of the bronchi. Symptoms include shortness of breath, expiratory (and inspiratory) wheeze, chest tightness, cough, air flow limitations (as seen in spirometry / peak expiratory flow rate (PEFR)).

Asthma reviews are structured reviews that occur on at least an annual basis and provide the healthcare professional conducting the review with the opportunity to assess how effectively the patient is managing their asthma in addition to evaluating their inhaler technique. It can also identify triggers, alert the practitioner to red flags and the need to adjust the patient's personal asthma plan and support self-management.

Case study: Jodie

You have been assigned to help with the asthma review clinic. The next patient to be seen is Jodie, a 28-year-old woman who has had asthma since childhood, which has generally been well controlled. She has suffered the occasional exacerbation of her asthma (although not warranting hospital admission). She is fully aware of her trigger (stress). For maintenance, she takes the preventer beclometasone (steroid) twice a day and reliever salbutamol as required.

She is currently on maternity leave since the birth of her first child 5 weeks ago. On arrival to the clinic, Jodie looks pale and tired. She admits that she has not been sleeping very well as she is the sole carer for her child (as her husband works long hours). She has no family or friends living nearby and feels isolated and alone. She has not been taking her beclometasone inhaler since the birth of her child. She is complaining that her chest feels 'tight' and she has a cough. She takes two puffs of her salbutamol inhaler approximately four times a day but this is not enough to relieve her symptoms.

Activity 3.3   Critical thinking

After reading the case study on Jodie, consider the following questions.

- What are Jodie's triggers?
- What are the red flags? Do you need to escalate and if so, why?
- What personal asthma action plan should be agreed with Jodie?
- Taking a holistic approach, what other factors/assessment/follow-up should be done?

An outline answer is given at the end of the chapter.

Case study: Maja

Your next patient is 53-year-old Maja, who has come in for a routine diabetic review.

From her records you establish that she has had bloods taken recently and her Hba$_{1c}$ has dramatically reduced. You are very pleased with this and anticipate that this will be good news for Maja. Her kidney function is slightly lower than last time. You decide to share this information with the nurse.

On examination you notice that Maja has dropped 2 stones (12.7 kg) in weight during the last 6 months. She states she has not been exercising, she feels good within herself and she has not noticed the weight loss. You ask if she has any concerns and she says she has none.

She has an appointment for her annual eye screening at the hospital next month and all her other observations are within normal parameters.

On further investigation you notice that Maja has a deep open wound on the bottom of her right foot. She states she has no pain when walking but that she does have sharp shooting pains when lying in bed.

Activity 3.4   Critical thinking

- What are your main concerns about Maja?
- What advice would you give Maja?
- Would you need to escalate any aspect of Maja's care? If so, to whom?
- Why is Maja only feeling pain when in bed at night?
- Why has Maja lost weight?
- Think about the Hba$_{1c}$; why is it low now?
- What is peripheral neuropathy?

An outline answer is given at the end of the chapter.

Case study: Gary

You have been asked to make a telephone call to Gary to relay his urgent blood results and also to inform him when his blood test needs to be repeated.

You call the mobile number recorded on the clinical system but a woman answers the phone. You explain who you are and where you are calling from and ask to speak to Gary. The woman replies that she is his wife and that you should let her know why you are calling and she will relay the message to her husband.

You advise the wife of your role and give her the details for her husband to call you back.

Gary returns your call and says you should have given his wife the full details.

You tell Gary his results and advise him he has to return in a month for another blood test. You book the blood test with him on the phone so he has the appointment in advance.

Activity 3.5   Critical thinking

- Were you wrong not to inform Gary's wife of his results in the first instance?
- What steps should you take to ensure that you are speaking to the correct person over the phone?
- Summarise your key learning points from this situation.
- How will you ensure that Gary does not miss the appointment booked to have his bloods retaken?

An outline answer is given at the end of the chapter.

Promotion of self-management

Today, policies and guidance on health and social care actively promote independence through patient-centred approaches. These methods recognise disparities within power relationships (between healthcare professionals and patients) and strive towards correcting them. However, it is acknowledged that in many cases there cannot be total equality in terms of power. Nonetheless, the empowerment and partnership model pays particular attention to the processes of participation and strongly advocates that the experiences of involvement should be meaningful for patients (i.e. that the patient should be actively involved throughout the whole process). Self-management within primary care is a key learning opportunity for you during a placement.

Person-centred approaches

Person-centred approaches to healthcare mean that individuals should be in control of their own health and care management. This type of system should concentrate on encouraging patient participation by respecting their autonomy and adopting a coordinated approach, in comparison to disjointed and isolated care. Service provision should also ensure that it is personalised and reactive to patients' requirements and beliefs.

Self-management has been defined as the process of learning and practising skills which enable individuals to manage their health condition on a day-to-day basis (Grady and Gough, 2014). This is achieved through individuals practising and adopting specific behaviours which are central to managing their condition, making informed decisions about care and engaging in healthy behaviours in order to reduce the physical and emotional impact of their illness (Grady and Gough, 2014).

From your placement you will realise that person-centred approaches to self-management are important to all patients, particularly to those with potential health problems and long-term conditions and the elderly. Patients taking an active role in their own care is central to effective quality care, enhancing outcomes and quality of life, as well as avoiding clinical deterioration.

Supported self-management

Supported self-management can provide patients with the assistance they require in order to reinforce and encourage the control they have over their own lives as well as reducing the restrictions inflicted on them by their present health or disability status. Supported self-management still views patients as active partners of care and not as passive recipients. This is the central philosophy of patient reviews and NHS Health Checks.

In order to be independent, it is imperative that the patient understands their role and the nature of the partnership between them and the healthcare professional. Firstly, an assessment should be conducted with the patient to determine where they are at in relation to gaining independence. For example, if an individual finds it difficult to participate with health issues or has complex problems, they are more likely to need more intensive support. There may, however, be many others who will be able to manage independently with minimal appropriate support when necessary.

If possible, take the opportunity to sit in on a few review consultations and note the different approaches of the staff in relation to promoting independence. Support should be provided in enabling patients to articulate clearly their requirements and to make a decision in relation to their preferences. This can be achieved by process of sharing information, collective decision making, goal setting and action planning. These care plans should be person-centred, holistic and comprising the complete array of health and social care requirements within the plan of care.

You will notice that, within the primary care setting, patients are encouraged to lead in their own care planning. As well as being individualised and personalised, care planning should have a structured education programme. This will include the provision of correct information, peer support, accessibility of healthcare professionals and physical, emotional, psychological and financial support when required. There are also a number of support programmes available, including volunteer-run general self-management education programmes (designed to develop patient knowledge, awareness, confidence, coping ability and social support) or through the use of interactive online programmes. These can increase the patient's knowledge, understanding, social support, health outcomes and health behaviours. Investigate what support services are available in your allocated placement.

Within your placement, you should observe that the emphasis within primary care is on adopting positive patient involvement in order to preserve health as much as possible. Care planning might include recommendations to non-traditional modes of support external to professional NHS services, e.g. those provided by voluntary organisations or community groups (which you may not see in a secondary care setting).

Another essential principle of patient involvement is that of family and carer involvement. This should be taken into consideration at all stages of care planning, decision making and care delivery. To retain and recognise patient autonomy, the patient must agree to the engagement of carers. Subject to informed consent (from the patient), information related to the care plan can be revealed to the carer.

Participation of families and carers can also help to increase the patient's self-awareness, self-confidence and insight into managing their health problems, lowering rates of relapse and hospital admissions and promoting rehabilitation of the patient. But do remember that some carers/family members themselves may periodically require input and support.

Participation

Those self-management programmes that are disease-specific (for example, asthma, diabetes) seem to be the most effective. This support can be in the form of psychosocial interventions, personalised coaching at the start of the patient's journey. In addition, the ability to monitor and evaluate one's behaviour and simplified medication administration (in terms of dosage) has achieved a decrease in service use and in cost as a result of the correct use of medications, fewer hospital admissions and unscheduled visits for specific diseases.

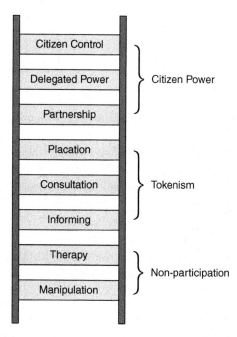

Figure 3.1 Ladder of Citizen Participation (Amstein, 1969).

The Ladder of Citizen Participation (Figure 3.1) shows the different levels of control from 'no control' (manipulation) to 'total control' (citizen control). This model can be used within primary care to demonstrate active or inactive patient and/or community engagement.

It is important to emphasise to patients the value of taking individual responsibility and control for their health. This includes adopting a healthier lifestyle, staying active, eating healthily, use of alcohol only in moderation and the avoidance of smoking. This approach not only benefits the patient (in terms of self-control and empowerment) but also healthcare professionals, the organisation and society in general.

As discussed, for such an approach to be successful, there needs to be an effective relationship and a good working partnership between the patient and healthcare professional. This should be based on honesty and trust, in addition to emphasising core values such as respect, partnership and equality (as far as possible) with relationships between service providers and service users and the need for adherence to monitoring and regular treatment, and involvement of family support.

Patient education should include a comprehensive programme of accessible and proactive care management including regular reviews. Flexibility and diversity in relation to the mode of contact to suit differing patients should be adopted, for example, consideration of email, telephone or video conferencing as opposed to in person. Patient self-managed support achieved through active telephone consultations that involve health coaching, motivational interviewing and psychosocial support can enhance self-assurance and self-management behaviours.

Factors that influence approaches to self-management and health promotion are patients' knowledge and understanding of their condition. As an NA, you will play a pivotal role in educating patients.

Student tip 3.1

During my studies I have learnt that preparation is key. I understand that I need to read through patient notes before the consultation and to prepare all the equipment I predict I will need.

This preparation meant that if a piece of equipment I needed was not available I would not look unprofessional and disorganised in front of the patient. Even better, I could spare the patient the trouble of travelling to the appointment only to be told that the equipment that I needed to perform their appointment was not available and therefore the appointment needed to be cancelled.

Reading the patient's notes beforehand enabled me to ask the nurse or other members of the team questions, such as on particular symptoms or medications.

Good preparation also saved me time during the consultation, giving patients an efficient and effective service.

Anya, first-year NA student

Chapter summary

This chapter has highlighted some of the key learning opportunities within the primary care setting. The main roles of the primary care nurse or NA have been discussed together with those of the MTD working within primary care.

Within the primary care environment there is a strong focus upon prevention of illness and promotion of health. This has been explored within the chapter with reference to the importance of NHS Health Checks and two of the main health reviews undertaken (diabetes and asthma). Aligned with this is the concept of self-management and self-management programmes. Even though you may not work in a primary care setting, it is a good idea to adopt some of the principles discussed within this chapter in relation to health promotion within your own workplace.

Activities: brief outline answers

Activity 3.2 Critical thinking

Kenneth's weight, BMI, waist circumference, family history and lack of activity put him at greater risk of diabetes. Request bloods for Hba_{1c} level and cholesterol. With Hba_{1c} check average blood sugar levels over the last 3 months. Raised cholesterol levels would indicate his risk of heart disease.

A urine sample to check albumin-to-creatinine ratio (ACR) would indicate kidney damage (a complication of diabetes). If diabetes is caught early, medication can stop the condition worsening.

Kenneth should be advised to lose weight through food and exercise. Refer him to a free/reduced-fee exercise programme if he needs assistance.

The NHS Health Check template only asks if more or less than five portions of fruit and vegetables are eaten per day. As an NA student you will need to go into more detail. An individual could be eating plenty of fruit and vegetables but also eating fried foods and foods with high sugar content. If necessary, you may need to suggest that the whole family make changes.

Referral to the diabetes prevention programme will depend on his Hba_{1c} result. This programme helps people implement real-life changes to their eating habits. It provides information about carbohydrates and how the body manages different food types. It also supports peer help groups.

Kenneth's alcohol intake is within normal limits, but if he reduces it further he could lose some weight with little effort. Some alcoholic beverages have a high fat content.

Other signs of diabetes are frequency of urination and issues with his feet or eyes, which should be assessed.

Give Kenneth patient information leaflets to read in his own time, as the amount of information given can be overwhelming.

Activity 3.3 Critical thinking

Stress has been mentioned as a trigger for Jodie's asthma. Her stress is unlikely to change while her personal life remains the same (caring for her baby with little support).

The fact that she has increased her usage of the reliever (salbutamol) yet still has symptoms (chest tightness, cough) is a red flag.

Discussion of a personal plan will need to include information about her newborn. As she does not have immediate support nearby and her husband works long hours, a social prescriber may help (refer the patient to local support groups). There may be local baby groups/mother-and-baby groups/baby massage available. Encourage Jodie to take walks with her baby, as sometimes this settles the baby and they are able to sleep well.

Explore the relationship between Jodie and her husband. Is he being supportive, or is he not involved? If possible, open up the possibility of her husband taking leave from work to support her for a few weeks and help her get rest and sleep.

As Jodie is under stress, this may affect her relationship with her newborn. Observe her interaction with her baby; assess whether a bond has been developed.

Baby checks should involve comparison of Jodie's weight before she had the baby to now (she should not be underweight so soon after giving birth).

Consider the possibility of anaemia (she looks pale and tired and is probably not eating very much or the right combination of foods). Depending upon Hb results, she may need a prescription for ferrous sulphate.

Make a review appointment for 2–3 weeks from now. Do not let Jodie arrange her own appointment later, as there is a risk that this will never happen. An afternoon appointment may be better as this will give her time to get ready without rushing.

Think about providing leaflets to do with the MDT (e.g. on post-natal depression and local centres for support for new parents).

Don't forget to print out an asthma action plan and give it to Jodie.

Activity 3.4 Critical thinking

Make sure you ask the nurse for help to assess the wound. If you are already proficient at wound assessment, give the nurse a clear report of the wound in order for them to plan care appropriately.

Look at the stage of the wound and think about appropriate dressing selection. There should be a local dressing formulary for you to adhere to. When choosing dressings, think about exudate management and infections in wounds.

Together with the nurse, create a care plan with clear red flags and dates to review. Book appointments for the patient in advance to ensure the wound is reviewed as planned.

Set clear next steps in case the wound becomes problematic, such as swabbing for infection and requesting antibiotics if needed or referring to a tissue viability nurse (TVN) for specialist help.

Look at the wound and assess the symptoms. Try to determine what type of wound it is. Is it a venous or arterial ulcer? Possibly ask the nurse or refer to the TVN for Doppler assessment.

Think about referral to a neurologist. Is the pain neuropathy? What can be done to relieve the symptoms?

Think about how the wound can cause a reduction in appetite, hence Maja's weight loss; this weight loss may not be healthy. Ask about any other symptoms; dig deeper to gain a holistic view of your patient's health condition. Consider the connection between weight loss and reduction in Hba_{1c}. If the reduced Hba_{1c} is because the wound is making the patient unwell, once the wound is healed will the food intake increase and then the Hba_{1c} too? The lifestyle advice you give can help the patient maintain a good weight and keep the Hba_{1c} down. Show the patient the correlation between weight loss and reduction in Hba_{1c} to encourage her that it can be done.

Peripheral neuropathy develops when nerves in the body's extremities, such as the hands, feet and arms, are damaged. The symptoms depend on which nerves are affected (NHS, 2019b). Symptoms include pins and needles, burning, shooting, stabbing pain, loss of balance or coordination and muscle weakness.

Activity 3.5 Critical thinking

Think about confidentiality. You need to ensure you are adhering to your practice confidential policy and procedures.

Make sure you check each patient's full name, date of birth and address before disclosing any aspect of their care. Many people have similar names and mistakes can easily be made if all credentials are not checked.

You can ask patients if they would like you to put a note on the system stating that they are happy for clinicians to share information about their care with a nominated person such as a partner or child.

To make sure that appointments are not missed, you can always follow up with a letter or text message to confirm the appointment details.

You can also add a pop-up message on his notes so that if any clinician has any interaction with him they can remind him of the appointment.

Another option is to have a list or spreadsheet of all patients who need following up and if they miss their appointments, make sure to contact them to rearrange.

Annotated further reading

The Queen's Nursing Institute (2015) *Transition to General Practice Nursing.* Available at: www.qni.org.uk/wp-content/uploads/2017/01/Transition-to-General-Practice-Nursing.pdf (accessed 16 June 2021).

Provides in-depth and comprehensive insight into primary care and the role of nursing within this setting.

Public Health England (2015) **NHS Health Check Competence Workshop Training Slides. Available at:** www.healthcheck.nhs.uk/commissioners-and-providers/national-guidance/ (accessed 8 July 2021).

The code of conduct within this workbook gives clear guidelines and boundaries for healthcare practitioners. The training slides contains useful links for learners and assessors alike.

Social care settings

Pam Hodge

NMC STANDARDS OF PROFICIENCY FOR REGISTERED NURSING ASSOCIATES (NMC, 2018A)

This chapter will address the following platforms and proficiencies:

Platform 2: Promoting health and preventing ill health

2.2   promote preventive health behaviours and provide information to support people to make informed choices to improve their mental, physical, behavioural health and wellbeing.

Platform 3: Provide and monitor care

3.5   work in partnership with people to encourage shared decision making, to support individuals, their families, and carers to manage their own care when appropriate.

3.6   demonstrate the knowledge, skills and ability to perform a range of nursing procedures and manage devices, to meet people's need for safe, effective and person-centred care.

Platform 5: Improving safety and quality of care

5.6   understand and act in line with local and national organisational frameworks, legislation, and regulations to report risks and implement actions as instructed, following up and escalating as required.

Platform 6: Contributing to integrated care

6.1   understand the roles of the different providers of health and care. Demonstrate the ability to work collaboratively and in partnership with professionals from different agencies in interdisciplinary teams.

6.3   demonstrate an understanding of the complexities of providing mental, cognitive, behavioural and physical care needs across a wide range of integrated care settings.

Introduction

This chapter will explore your practice learning role as an NA student in social care settings. For your practice learning you require a registered nurse or NA to meet the Standards for Student Supervision and Assessment (NMC, 2018c), as explored in Chapter 2. It may surprise you to learn that 36,000 registered nurses represent 44.4% of all registered professionals working in adult social care (Skills for Care, 2020), and that 33,000 of these work in care homes with nursing care.

There are four main sections in this chapter outlining the learning you can expect to gain from a social care placement:

1. the integration of health and social care – putting the service user first
2. interprofessional working, including your role as an NA student
3. effective communication, including health promotion
4. awareness of the regulations and clinical governance in the social care sector

These provide the opportunity to gain valuable knowledge, experience and skills that you can develop and apply in other care settings.

What is social care?

Undertake Activity 4.1 to establish what you already understand by the term "social care".

Activity 4.1   Critical thinking

Note down your thoughts on the following questions:

- What do we mean by social care?
- Who can be supported by social care?

You can review your answers to this activity as we consider social care.
   As this activity is based on your own reflection, there is no outline answer at the end of the chapter.

Formal definitions of social care vary; however, they have similar components, which we will now explore. A dictionary definition is a useful starting point (OED, 2021):

"Social care is the provision by society of what is necessary for the health and welfare of a person or group of people"

The National Health Service and Community Care Act (Government, 1990) provides a more specific set of criteria, including the provision of social work, personal care, protection or social support services to children or adults in need or at risk, or adults with needs arising from illness, disability, old age or poverty.
   The Social Care Institute for Excellence (SCIE, 2015) develop these definitions and state that social care:

"may have one or more of the following aims:

- to protect service users,
- to preserve or advance physical or mental health,
- to promote independence and social inclusion,
- to improve opportunities and life chances,
- to strengthen families and protect human rights in relation to people's social needs".

Social care is therefore used as an umbrella term for many roles and settings which support vulnerable people. This could include people of all age ranges in settings which are residential, domiciliary, day services or community-based, including people with learning disabilities or mental ill health.

Learning from social care practice: integration of health and social care

In 2019 the Department of Health became the Department of Health and Social Care. This occurred after a series of important reviews and strategic planning into the best way to support people who require care in the community. This included the *Five Year Forward View* (NHS England, 2014) and subsequent *Next Steps* (NHS England, 2017), and the NHS *Long-Term Plan* (NHS England, 2019), highlighting how the NHS and social care need to work together to avoid unnecessary admissions to hospital and facilitate early discharge from acute care.

The Care Quality Commission have emphasised the need for integrated working, advising:

> The way we plan, commission and deliver health and care must be shaped by the experience of dealing with a national health emergency, which has shown so very clearly how interdependent health and care truly are.

(CQC, 2020)

Integrated care systems are now evolving to strengthen integrated working: "instead of working independently every part of the NHS, public health and social care system should continue to seek out ways to connect, communicate and collaborate so that the health and care needs of people are met" (DoHSC, 2021, p. 10). Care homes with nursing care are one of the practice areas where this integration is most visible and supports the agenda of care closer to home (Kings Fund, 2018).

We will now look at this in context in the following case study.

Case study: Rokaya

Rokaya (70 years old) was admitted to hospital with a fractured hip. She fell whilst struggling to carry her grocery shopping home, where she lives alone.

Whilst in hospital Rokaya was diagnosed with hypertension and type 2 diabetes, which can be managed with dietary changes. Rokaya is prescribed valsartan; the dose is being monitored and titrated.

Rokaya has capacity and has agreed that she will require a short stay in a care home with nursing care to facilitate her recovery and to assess the type of care package she will require in the future. This type of care is commonly referred to as the 'discharge to assess' pathway.

Health and social care services will need to work together effectively; including undertaking assessments to ensure Rokaya's care needs are met and there is a seamless transition from hospital to care home.

Rokaya is discharged to the care home with a 7-day prescription and follow-up appointments.

Now consider Activity 4.2 to relate this case study to your practice learning.

Activity 4.2   Critical thinking

You accompany the registered nurse to meet with Rokaya in hospital to undertake an assessment to determine whether your care home can meet Rokaya's needs.

- What type of support will Rokaya require?
- What are your key considerations when undertaking this holistic assessment?

(Continued)

(Continued)

- How will you actively involve Rokaya in the assessment process?
- How does this scenario help you to consider integrated health and social care?

An outline answer is given at the end of the chapter.

Care homes have different specialisms and skills; not all will meet every person's holistic needs. Care homes offer several different services, beyond the 'discharge to assess'; some people attend for brief or respite periods, whereas others call the care home their home for many months or years. This is a key learning point for you during a social care placement. It is worth remembering that you are working in the person's home and may develop a working relationship over an extended period. Your need to be approachable and accommodating must be balanced with your need for ongoing professionalism. This longer-term working will also allow you and service users to develop truly holistic care plans, including personal preferences and goal setting. One example of this is the advanced care plan.

> Advance care planning is a process that supports adults at any age or stage of health in understanding and sharing their personal values, life goals, and preferences regarding future medical care. The goal of advance care planning is to help ensure that people receive medical care that is consistent with their values, goals and preferences during serious and chronic illness.
>
> International Consensus Definition of Advance Care Planning
> (Sudore et al., 2017).

The UK health and social care systems are under increasing pressure to meet changing population needs, with 100% increase in the number of people aged 85 years or older expected in the next 20 years (Skills for Care, 2020). Service users in need of care home support are experiencing multiple morbidities with complex care needs and require staff teams whose skills match this need (DoHSC, 2021). The co-morbidities may be acute or, increasingly, involve multiple long-term conditions.

The NA qualification is well suited to care home working, being generic and incorporating caring for all ages and multiple morbidities (NHS Employers, 2019). All the England NA Practice Assessment Document (PAD) (PLPLG, 2019) proficiencies can be completed in care homes, subject to service user need at any given time. A placement in a care home can support you to meet the Standards of Proficiency for Registered Nursing Associates (NMC, 2018a).

Learning from social care practice: interprofessional working

Care homes are nurse-led services. This requires a high level of clinical skill to manage the complexity of care needs. One of these skills is knowing when and how to liaise with other healthcare professionals.

You will be working with people with dementia in many care settings, including social care. In the UK, 5.2% of the population under 65 years have a diagnosis of a type of dementia. This rises to 20% for 85–89-year-olds (Dementia Statistics, 2021) with some form of cognitive decline; that is, a decline of brain functioning related to memory, problem solving, learning new skills and retaining new information. Short-term memory loss is most common and an early indicator for many brain function changes.

However, 'Dementia is not only about memory loss. It can also affect the way you speak, think, feel and behave' (NHS, 2020).

You will have heard the umbrella term of dementia frequently used. Activity 4.3 asks you to undertake some research to identify common types of dementia and how they occur.

Activity 4.3   Evidence-based practice

Look up the causes and presentations associated with the following types of dementia:

- Alzheimer's
- Vascular dementia
- Lewy body
- Frontotemporal dementia

An outline answer is given at the end of the chapter.

After completing Activity 4.3 you will have discovered that there are a range of causes, symptoms and presentations related to organic cognitive decline. The people that you will be caring for will, therefore, have complex care needs which may fluctuate.

Meeting service users' holistic needs requires an MDT approach. We will explore this in the following case study.

Case study: John

John (55 years old) has frontotemporal dementia. John is well liked, approachable and has a good sense of humour. John is a retired English teacher who enjoys watching rugby and reading.

Susie, John's wife, noticed a change approximately 3 years ago; John was less 'engaged', his face was less expressive and he sometimes appeared lost for words. The GP undertook some physical health tests including kidney and liver function tests to find possible causes for the change, including a trial for 6 months on antidepressants, but found nothing.

Susie noticed further changes in John's presentation. Though usually calm, John was now quick to anger and was less able to empathise with others. His family also

(Continued)

(Continued)

reported behaviour that was out of character; he was not reading any more and he used to water the garden repeatedly, no matter what time of day or night.

The GP spoke with John, who agreed to meet with a psychologist based in the GP practice in the Improving Access to Psychological therapies (IAPT) service. As part of this assessment, the psychologist undertook a Mini Mental State Exam (MMSE). The assessment showed some cognitive decline; however, the most noticeable observation was that John struggled to reply, being hesitant and slow and providing answers unrelated to the questions. He had aphasia. At times John became frustrated and angry with himself that he could not answer correctly.

John was referred to a specialist old age psychiatrist who requested a positron emission tomography (PET) scan at the local hospital to further investigate the causes of John's condition. This resulted in evidence of degeneration in the brain. Piecing this together with all the other information, John was diagnosed with frontotemporal dementia.

John lost some of his muscle strength and motor skills as his dementia progressed. The muscle atrophy resulted in progressive dysphagia and changes to his gait. Susie found it increasingly challenging to care for John. In discussion with the GP and social work team, it was agreed that John required care home with nursing care support.

A range of professionals had supported John in the community, including a daily care home package. Once at the care home the MDT expanded further as John's dementia progressed and his care needs increased.

Now you have been introduced to John we will think about the wider MDT who will support John to meet his complex needs.

At the point of admission, you will be involved in developing a holistic person-centred care plan with John and be involved in making referrals to the MDT. We will explore some of the professionals you may work with in a social care setting in Activity 4.4.

Activity 4.4 Evidence-based practice

After reading the case study about John, identify his care needs, including his integrated physical, mental, social and behavioural needs.

Identify who you will involve in John's care to support particular aspects of care. For example, GP to review John's overall health needs and consider medication reviews if required.

An outline answer is given at the end of the chapter.

With so many professionals involved in the care of one person, you will see that effective communication strategies with the wider MDT are key areas of learning in a social care placement. There will be MDT meetings, in person, virtually or via phone calls and you will need to document accurately the discussions adjusting care plans as needed, and update your care home colleagues to implement any changes to the care plan. As an NA student you will also be expected to ensure these changes are implemented in practice, demonstrating part of your leadership role, including being aware of your own limitations and when to escalate to ensure service user safety as per the NMC Code (NMC, 2018d). Working with other professionals in this way is another key learning point from a social care placement.

Learning from social care practice: effective communication

'Communication is a multi-dimensional, multi-factorial phenomenon and a dynamic, complex process, closely related to the environment in which an individual's experiences are shared' (Wanko Keutchafo et al., 2020, p. 1). This definition encompasses various aspects which make effective communication key to your role, and importantly contextualise it to the specific practice area.

When you think of communication, perhaps you consider verbal or written communication. What about the array of non-verbal communications (NVC)? Research into the NVC adopted with older people in care settings has shown extensive reliance on this type of communication (Wanko Keutchafo et al., 2020). This makes sense when you think the person may have an altered ability to process information; for example, if they have dementia, neurological diversity or a sensory impairment which may challenge comprehension.

NVC skills include the use of silence, the art of active listening, proxemics (position of yourself to the person), haptics (appropriate touch), tone of speech, kinesics (movements or gestures) and any form of written or visual communication.

Obtaining consent to undertake care is fundamental. In social care you will be working with the most vulnerable people, some of whom will have fluctuating capacity, and you will need to adopt an advocacy role (NMC, 2018d). We will explore effective communication within the following case study.

Case study: Ngozi

Ngozi (30 years old) has a diagnosis of moderate learning disability and impaired hearing in her left ear. Ngozi enjoys working in a local print shop and the social aspects of her job. She lives in specialist supported accommodation.

The NA who works with her has noticed that Ngozi has not engaged in the weekly community meetings and appears to be isolating herself, sometimes, unusually for Ngozi, sleeping in the day.

Ngozi is agreeable to discussing her problems with the NA and identifies that she feels tired all the time and worries that she is not well. After discussion Ngozi agrees to attend an appointment with the practice nurse whom Ngozi knows well and that the NA can accompany her to this meeting.

(Continued)

(Continued)

The practice nurse takes a history from Ngozi who describes feeling tired all the time since her last birthday (3 months ago). The practice nurse explains that she will need to take a blood test and then they will talk again. Ngozi understands as she has annual blood tests as part of her review and associates the practice nurse with this check.

The NA accompanies Ngozi to see the practice nurse again. The practice nurse reports that Ngozi's haemoglobin reading is low at 110 g/L (normal range for a female: 115–165 g/L; NICE, 2018b). Initially, Ngozi does not understand what is said and becomes anxious. The NA agrees to explain the concern to Ngozi and that she has options regarding her treatment.

The NA is aware of Ngozi's hearing impairment and makes sure that she sits on the right side of Ngozi. She uses short sentences and a calm tone to try and explain the low iron in the blood. Ngozi struggles to understand the verbal communication.

The NA was prepared for this and has printed an easy-read booklet on anaemia to support Ngozi, who finds the pictures and explanations easier to follow. Ngozi feels less anxious.

The practice nurse and NA need to ensure that Ngozi has understood the issue and the NA asks Ngozi to explain her understanding. Ngozi reports that she has too little iron and needs more to stop feeling tired all the time and wants to not feel tired.

There is a choice of treatments available, including a vitamin B_{12} intramuscular injection regularly, a change of diet to include more iron-rich foods, and, if needed, ferrous sulphate tablets in the future.

The NA has made sure that she has enough time to spend with Ngozi upon returning to the accommodation and they discuss the options together. Health education and promotion are discussed in terms of adding more iron-rich foods into Ngozi's diet. Ngozi develops a pictorial list with the NA for when she goes shopping. Ngozi also understands that the vitamin B_{12} injection could help boost her ability to produce iron and agrees to this intervention.

The NA orders the medication to administer. Ngozi agrees to return for another blood test in 3 months to review with the practice nurse.

The NA updates the care notes and care plan, advising colleagues of the changes.

People in social care settings link with primary care services on a regular basis and it is necessary to have effective communication between the services (when consent is given). In this scenario the NA was able to support Ngozi by accompanying and ensuring the information was clear to Ngozi and those at the supported accommodation to help Ngozi manage her health.

Activity 4.5 asks you to critique the case study and relate it to your practice.

Activity 4.5   Critical thinking

Please consider the case study of Ngozi.

- Thinking about the communication strategies used by the NA, what did she do well?
- How could this interaction have been enhanced?
- How did the NA ensure Ngozi understood?
- Did Ngozi demonstrate capacity to make an informed choice about her care? How?
- How will you use this scenario to inform your own practice?

An outline answer is given at the end of the chapter.

As an NA student you may be employed in an NHS Trust. Not all students will have a social care placement; however, developing a good knowledge of social care can support your understanding of the integrated systems. This will provide you with valuable insight into the relationships and communication strategies between practice areas. This knowledge will help you ensure a smooth transition for the service user from hospital discharge to a care home, or vice versa if you are employed in social care.

There are several processes to support this communication, including the Red Bag, where service user information and belongings, including medications, are contained and stay with the person on their journey around the hospital. This means information can be viewed, reviewed and returned to the care home with any changes to care plans and medication. Key information stays with the service user and effective communication and subsequent care can be achieved – an example of prioritising the person (NMC, 2018d). There may be other local initiatives in your placement area for you to locate and reflect upon.

Learning from social care practice: regulation and governance

Working in social care settings is different to working in the NHS. Social care settings are usually independently run, may be part of a larger company and only 6% of social care is NHS- or state-owned (CQC, 2020). Social care funding also differs, with some service users assessed as having to contribute towards their care, as opposed to NHS care that is funded by the Department of Health and Social Care. For your practice learning, it will be important to consider that those in social care settings may well be, at least partially, self-funding elements of their care.

With many different organisations providing care, with different levels of expertise, the sector needs to be regulated to ensure standardised best quality of care is provided. Activity 4.6 explores your understanding of social care sector regulation.

Activity 4.6   Research

Please answer the following questions:

- Who are the Care Quality Commission (CQC)?
- What are the five inspection areas?
- What do the award levels mean in practice?
- How can these domains be demonstrated as met in your practice area?

An outline answer is given at the end of the chapter.

The CQC are a national independent body set up to regulate health and social care. Inspections are carried out approximately every 2 years if there are no concerns, although more often if there are concerns or complaints. Inspection visits may be planned or unannounced. The whole practice area is audited, including speaking with service users, families and staff. The five domain areas are graded and incorporated into the report, posted online and available to the public. The CQC as regulator also produce best-practice guides to follow, as well as the yearly State of Care report which gives an overview of the health and social care system in England. The CQC have the power to limit care activity in practice areas or, in extreme circumstances where there are serious concerns, to close areas.

Student tip 4.1

For social care settings I found it helpful to go to the CQC website and search for the placement area. You will be able to find out key information, such as the licensed range of support and care provided on the main page. There are also inspection summaries to read as well as the whole document.

This can help you orientate to the area, consider the service user cohort, formulate your learning objective and guide your wider reading.

Jordache, Year 2 NA student

Social care settings, whilst independently run, will also be working towards, or have achieved, nationally recognised standards, for example the Gold Standards Framework in Care Homes (see annotated links at the end of the chapter), which relates to end-of-life care.

You can demonstrate your proactive learning by asking which frameworks are used in your practice area and how you can be involved. For example, NA students in social care settings are leading on a variety of initiatives to feed into the wider overall package of clinical governance, defined as 'activities that help sustain and improve high standards of patient care' (RCN, 2021). Examples include becoming manual handling lead; being responsible for the implementation and audit of the Significant 7 protocol (see annotated reading list); and oral care champion in the practice area and part of a wider national network to inform best practice. NA students are taking on training responsibilities, as well as championing and auditing the care provision; you will be an integral part of the team.

Chapter summary

In social care, you will have the opportunity to support vulnerable people with complex care needs at different stages in their journey and become familiar with the MDT in the community.

Social care placements, as well as offering the opportunity to potentially complete your NA PAD proficiencies, can provide you with valuable experience of working with people over a longer period, building therapeutic relationships and developing truly holistic care plans.

Social care placements allow you to experience the integration of health and social care in action.

Social care is a huge topic and practice area. This book cannot attempt to cover all aspects of social care, but rather is an introduction to working and learning in social care. There are links to wider reading at the end of this chapter to guide you in developing your knowledge.

To review your learning from this chapter please undertake Activity 4.7.

Activity 4.7   Reflection

How has your understanding of social care altered because of reading this chapter? (Consider your prior knowledge/understanding, what you have learnt, and what you need to find out more about.)

As this answer is based on your own reflection, there is no outline answer at the end of the chapter.

Activities: brief outline answers

Activity 4.2 Critical thinking

Rokaya will need support in the following areas:

- to transition from hospital to the care home and regain increased independence and confidence

- physiotherapy to support with mobilising and exercise advice to recover from the fracture.
- medication monitoring and review for the hypertension, as well as health promotion strategies
- blood / glucose monitoring and diabetes health education and advice, including on special dietary requirements

Key considerations when undertaking this holistic assessment are that Rokaya should be aware of the processes involved and her options. The following areas of the NMC Code (2018d) are relevant:

- Prioritise the person: Rokaya's wishes and dignity need to be maintained, respecting Rokaya as an individual with holistic needs, including biological, psychological, social, cultural, behavioural and spiritual.
- Practise effectively: evidence-based practice should be maintained; regular relevant training needs to be undertaken; there is clear communication with Rokaya and the wider MDT; and all the relevant assessment information is collated, documented and reviewed.
- Preserve safety: does the care home team offer all the care Rokaya will require on site or have access to the wider MDT? Does the team have the correct skills mix?

To actively involve Rokaya in the assessment process, you should discuss with Rokaya her understanding of her care needs and how these can be met in the care home; establish what Rokaya would identify as important to her and her recovery goals; whom she may wish to involve in her care – for example, any family members; answer any questions and offer her a visit, whether virtual or physical, as soon as possible. Make it clear to Rokaya she does not have to agree to move to the care home; it is her choice.

This scenario helps us to consider integrated health and social care in the context that, for Rokaya to have a seamless care journey, both the acute Trust and the social care provider, the care home, need to work together to ensure that Rokaya's needs are met in their assessments and agreements. By undertaking this collaborative working, the NHS is supported to facilitate Rokaya's early release from hospital, freeing space to care for others, and the care home are clear they can meet Rokaya's care and support needs and fill a vacancy. Both health and social care gain and Rokaya has a seamless care experience.

Activity 4.3 Evidence-based practice

- Alzheimer's: the most common cause of dementia

Not all causes of Alzheimer's dementia are known, but some relate to three gene mutations. The condition is probably congenital, and is transmitted from parent to child. The disease is characterised by tangles of fibrous protein and plaques (clumps of protein) in the brain, potentially damaging healthy neurons and their pathways.

- Vascular dementia: the second most common type of dementia

Vascular dementia is caused by blood supply to the brain. This type of dementia may be the result of a stroke or other vascular event. 'The most common symptoms of vascular dementia include difficulties with problem-solving, slowed thinking, focus and organization. These tend to be more noticeable than memory loss' (Mayo Clinic, 2020).

- Lewy body: a common progressive dementia

    Lewy bodies are the clumps of protein found in the brain of patients with this condition. Lewy body dementia is characterised by parkinsonian movements, difficulty in maintaining focus or attention and commonly visual hallucinations, which may be distressing.

- Frontotemporal dementia: commonly occurs in those under 65 years old

    Frontotemporal dementia is difficult to diagnose. It is caused by the degeneration of nerve cells in the front and temporal lobe areas of the brain; these areas affect language, behaviour and personality.

Activity 4.4 Evidence-based practice

The following professionals and individuals may be involved in John's care:

- physiotherapist: to support John to maintain muscle integrity if possible and counteract the atrophy the dementia will cause
- occupational therapist: to work with John to support him to undertake activities, perhaps with physical aids
- speech and language therapist: to support the care home team with specialist advice and planning as John struggles with language (aphasia); also, as his condition worsens, John may require support to eat due to muscle atrophy and related dysphagia
- activities coordinator: to work with John and the occupational therapist to ensure John is included in occupying his time, in a way which is manageable for him, if wanted
- community mental health nurse: to support John with his mental wellbeing and review his mental state
- tissue viability nurse: as John's muscle atrophy intensifies, he may require specialist support to maintain skin integrity
- palliative care team: as John approaches the end of his life, the palliative care team may work with the care home nursing and NA team to ensure John is comfortable and his wishes are respected
- social worker: the social worker is involved to access the care home funding, and is involved with Mental Capacity Act (Department of Health, 2005) testing and any related deprivation of liberty safeguards that are enacted. The social worker may also support with carers assessments for Susie.

- family members: if John is able to consent to his family being involved in his care, they may be integral to the plan to comfort John at times of distress, being aware of John's preferences and interests to support the care home team to engage John with activities. For example, whilst John may not be able to engage in conversation as he used to or read, he might enjoy listening to the news or to his favourite authors' audio-recorded novels

Activity 4.5 Critical thinking

- Thinking about the communication strategies used by the NA, what did she do well?

Your opinions will be individual. However, you may have included the following points: ensuring she had time to spend with Ngozi to have the conversation and support her needs; good positioning to ensure Ngozi could hear well; reacting to Ngozi's anxiety in a calm manner; using more than one method of information sharing – verbal, easy-read, picture shopping list; having a back-up support plan to ensure Ngozi was made to feel valued; using short sentences which are less confusing; using a language level that Ngozi understands; asking Ngozi to confirm what she had understood; empowering Ngozi to make decisions about her care.

- How could this interaction have been enhanced?

Again, you will have your own opinions, but they may include the following. The NA had foreshadowed that Ngozi would find the verbal communication challenging; perhaps using the easy-read from the beginning would have been better, reducing Ngozi's anxiety and preventing her from feeling that she did not understand; the NA could have asked Ngozi how she would like to have this information shared – perhaps Ngozi has a preferred method she knows works well for her? There are other ways the information could have been shared; for example, using a simple diagram or video showing iron in the blood.

- How did the NA ensure Ngozi understood?

The NA asked Ngozi to explain to the NA what she understood was meant by having a low iron count.

- Did Ngozi demonstrate capacity to make an informed choice about her care? How?

'A person must be assumed to have capacity unless it is established that he lacks capacity' (Principle 1, section 1(2), Mental Capacity Act, 2005) (Department of Health, 2005). The Mental Capacity Act tells us there are four factors in the decision matrix when assessing capacity: understanding the information relevant to the decision; retaining that information; weighing up that information in terms of positives and negatives of undertaking/not undertaking the action; and being able to communicate that decision. In Ngozi's case, she demonstrated an understanding of the information, retained the information to be able to decide, reported that if she didn't act she might stay tired all the time and did not wish this to happen, and she was able to communicate this to the NA.

- How will you use this scenario to inform your own practice?

An answer is not provided as this will be specific to your learning.

Activity 4.6 Research

- Who are the Care Quality Commission?

This is answered within the chapter; more information can be found here: www.cqc.org.uk/about-us/our-purpose-role/who-we-are

- What are the five inspection areas?

Safe; effective; caring; responsive; well led.

- What do the inspection levels mean in practice?

Outstanding: the service is performing exceptionally well
Good (green): the service is performing well and meeting our expectations
Requires improvement (amber): the service isn't performing as well as it should and we have told the service how it must improve
Inadequate (red): the service is performing badly and we've taken enforcement action against the provider of the service
No rating/under appeal/rating suspended (grey): there are some services which we can't rate, while some might be under appeal from the provider. Suspended ratings are being reviewed by us and will be published soon

(CQC, 2021: www.cqc.org.uk/location/1-105863325/inspection-summary#icon-keys)

- How can these domains be demonstrated as met in your practice area?

The answer to this question will be specific to your practice area.

Annotated further reading

NHS England (n.d.) *Quick Guide: Discharge to Access.* Available at: www.nhs. uk/nhsengland/keogh-review/documents/quick-guides/quick-guide-discharge-to-access.pdf (accessed 16 June 2021).

An overview of the 'discharge to assess' definitions, process, and pathways.

Mughal, A.F. (2014) Understanding and using the Mental Capacity Act. *Nursing Times*, 110(21): 16–18.

This is an article on the Mental Capacity Act (2005), which is clear to follow.

QNI (2018) *Transition to Care Home Nursing*. Available at: www.qni.org.uk/nursing-in-the-community/transition-community-nursing/care-home-nursing/ (accessed 6 July 2021).

This outlines the role of the nurse in care homes.

Annotated useful websites

To find out more about the Red Bag scheme: https://healthinnovationnetwork.com/projects/transfer-of-care-the-red-bag-project-in-care-homes/

To find out more about the Significant 7 tool: www.nelft.nhs.uk/significant-7/

To find out more about the Gold Standards Framework: www.goldstandardsframework.org.uk/

Royal College of Nursing – Care Home Journey: www.rcn.org.uk/clinical-topics/older-people/professional-resources/care-home-journey

Social Care Institute of Excellence. Use of Deprivation of Liberty Safeguards in Care and Nursing Homes: www.scie.org.uk/mca/dols/practice/care-home

Care England – Pilot Study: details meaningful activities with people experiencing dementia: http://paper.uscip.us/ajad/AJAD.2015.1003.pdf

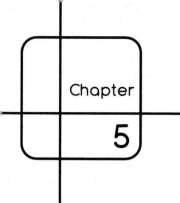

Mental health settings

Adrian Jugdoyl and
Marion Taylor

(Continued)

Platform 6: Contributing to integrated care

At the point of registration, the nursing associate will be able to:

6.1 understand the roles of the different providers of health and care. Demonstrate the ability to work collaboratively and in partnership with professionals from different agencies in interdisciplinary teams.

6.2 understand and explore the challenges of providing safe nursing care for people with complex co-morbidities and complex care needs.

6.3 demonstrate an understanding of the complexities of providing mental, cognitive, behavioural and physical care needs across a wide range of integrated care settings.

Chapter aims

After reading this chapter, you will be able to:

- discuss the range of placement settings available within Mental Health (MH) settings.
- identify the learning opportunities which can be gained from undertaking a placement within a variety of MH settings which can be transferred to other areas of practice.
- identify a range of communication techniques used across MH settings when caring for complex service user needs which can be used in other settings.
- identify the variety of treatments within MH and how such knowledge can be utilised as a transferable skill.
- understand factors that influence MH and wellbeing.

Introduction

The UK Government report *No Health Without Mental Health* (UK Government, 2011) recognises that promoting good MH and providing early interventions could improve healthcare outcomes for the future. As a Nursing Associate (NA) student undertaking a placement within MH settings, you will be exposed to service users with a range of MH issues. Therefore, having an understanding of how MH impacts physical health is vital. A specific MH placement may not be available for all students, but it is important to recognise that you may have opportunities to care for patients with MH care needs in other settings such as accident and emergency, acute medical wards or in elderly care wards. This chapter will support your learning for those situations, as well as specific MH placements.

This chapter will begin by discussing the importance of effective communication within MH care and identifying an effective technique used within MH to enhance communication. Following this, the range of MH care settings accessed by service users will be discussed, exploring the key concepts of working with service users in such settings. There are numerous MH settings that range from the community and home care settings to secure inpatient units (sometimes known as inservice user units). MH care crosses all ages, genders and cultures, and can present many challenges. This chapter will include identifying opportunities for interprofessional working and learning and transferable skills to support MH service users in all settings. The term 'service user' is used in most MH settings rather than patient, and this term is therefore used within this chapter. One common exception is 'inpatient' and 'outpatient' units or facilities.

Developing your communication skills

When working within an MH setting, sensitive situations often arise where effective communication is essential. You will learn to adapt your communication skills to elicit information for service users who may initially be reluctant to share this. You will build your confidence in communicating effectively with service users to gather information to support their condition and treatment (Servellen and Maram, 2020). Healthcare professionals must be equipped to communicate and treat service users with MH conditions in various settings. Therefore, an MH placement will provide you with the opportunity to develop these transferable communication skills. These skills do however take time to develop, and you may observe these but not always be able to put them into practice as an NA student yourself.

Providing treatment for those expressing mental stress is very demanding and requires high-level communication. Behaviours such as aggression, confusion or evidence of self-harm can be challenging for healthcare professionals, and this is something you will experience when undertaking an MH placement. Working within an MH setting where service users are being supported and treated allows you to respond to these behaviours in a supported environment effectively. Stigma of MH is often a barrier to providing acceptable healthcare activity (Knaak et al., 2017). An MH setting provides you with exposure to conditions and treatments that are often misunderstood. You will have the opportunity to develop a sound knowledge base about such conditions and treatments.

Activity 5.1   Reflection

As mentioned above, there is often a stigma applied to MH care and conditions. In order to appreciate the impact this may have, it is worth considering the following questions:

- Consider how many times in the past month you have used words that could be seen as stigmatising to service users. What other words could you have used that may be more acceptable?
- Have you ever been a service user or carer of a service user and felt that you were not being listened to?

As this is based on your own reflection, there is no outline answer for this activity.

Having completed Activity 5.1 we will explore communication in difficult circumstances further. Breaking bad news or explaining challenges ahead is an integral part of healthcare. Developing an effective professional relationship with service users and families is vital to supporting service users with the condition. When communication is handled poorly, this can have a long-term detrimental effect on the service user and their family members. Service users with MH conditions may find communication difficult and may exhibit body language that presents a barrier to open communication; for example, poor eye contact. MH settings offer you a wide range of service users and families with differing communication skills, styles and needs.

Motivational interviewing is a communication technique often used across healthcare settings, and in particular within MH. Simper et al. (2017) identified motivational interviewing as person-centred, offering an opportunity for collaboration between healthcare practitioners and service users. You may be able to observe this technique used in practice with your practice assessor (PA) or practice supervisor (PS), who will be useful role models of this. Motivational interviewing techniques are commonly abbreviated to OARS (open questions, affirmations, reflective listening and summarising). Using the acronym OARS will help in a variety of settings and allow for more effective communications. It is therefore a useful skill you may develop in an MH setting wihich you can transfer to other areas of practice. OARS is explained further as follows.

Open questions

Asking open questions allows people to have an open discussion; it removes yes–no answers and allows for conversation to remain general.

An example of a closed question would be: are things better than they were before? This type of question leads predominantly to a yes or no response.

On the other hand, an example of an open question would be: 'So, I know we have not spoken for a while. How have things been since we last met?' This type of question moves away from a yes or no answer.

Affirmations

This means expressing interest and understanding. This will help manage conflict and authenticity in the conversation by being genuine and acknowledging that experiences can be complex or challenging. Recognising things are difficult will show that you are engaged.

Reflective listening

Reflective listening is also used to show empathy, interest and understanding to you, the listener; it also requires concentration as conversations can become very abrupt and short if the service user does not feel as if they are being listened to.

Summarising

Summarising reinforces what has been said, confirms that you have been listening and aids in drawing conclusions that have been agreed upon.

For more information on motivational interviewing in the context of MH, please see Miller and Rollnick (2013).

Activity 5.2   Reflection

Having looked at motivational interviewing principles as an effective communication technique used in MH, let us now reflect on how delivering bad news to a service user could be improved. The bad news could be a diagnosis which will require long-term management, an alternative medication requirement or that a transfer to a different unit is needed. You will also be aware of 'bad news' in other settings which may relate to diagnosis or prognosis.

Reflect on how you have seen bad news being communicated to service users.

- How could this be improved?
- What fundamental principles would the service user want?
- Does this include empathy, honesty, transparency and a plan?
- How could you support a service user if they have recently received bad news?

An outline answer is given at the end of the chapter.

Learning from mental health care settings

Whilst the majority of MH care is delivered in the community setting, there are other settings where it can be delivered and which are supported by nurses and NAs trained in MH care. These include:

- home (in a service user's own home)
- community clinics
- substance misuse services (in hospital and the community)
- acute hospitals
- MH hospitals and inpatient facilities such as the forensic care unit
- prison
- specialist rehabilitation services
- other 'places of safety' (for example, Section 136 suites)

A Section 136 suite is a facility for people whom the Police detain under Section 136 of the Mental Health Act. It provides a 'place of safety' whilst potential MH needs are assessed under the Mental Health Act (1983) and any necessary arrangements made for ongoing care. The process of sectioning a service user is explored later within this chapter.

Most local hospitals or Clinical Commissioning Groups (CCGs) will include the above services and may offer opportunities for you to attend during your placement in MH. In some MH settings a uniform is not worn, but a dress code is followed. You will be advised on the policy for your placement area in advance. In community settings, there is the opportunity to meet people and talk and listen to them about their health. However, medication is not generally administered within the community. An opportunity to work with an independent nurse prescriber may be provided during your programme; this is an excellent opportunity to understand better this specialised route of nursing care and how it works alongside the medical prescribing routes. You may also have the opportunity to experience the pharmacy side of dispensing medication under supervision.

Mental health treatments

Depending on the MH setting, the treatments offered will vary. It is essential to recognise that service users presenting in one setting may be better treated in another setting as their MH condition evolves. MH treatments can broadly be separated into three groups:

1. talking therapies
2. medication
3. other, e.g. alcohol detoxification

It is important to recognise that a combination of all the different types of treatments can be delivered in some settings, particularly inpatient MH facilities.

We will now explore communication, specifically talking therapies, starting with an activity.

Activity 5.3   Evidence-based practice

Before learning about how talking therapies are used to support service users with MH, undertake a review of your own knowledge and literature search to identify some MH conditions that you think may be supported by talking therapies.

An outline answer is given at the end of the chapter.

Talking therapies

Talking therapies are generally delivered in the community setting by the local Improving Access to Psychological Therapies (IAPT) service. Talking therapies are psychological treatments for common mental and emotional disorders like stress, anxiety and depression. Generally, across England, service users can self-refer to their local IAPT service to access talking therapies. Service users assessed as having mild to moderate common MH disorders are generally considered suitable for community-based treatment through IAPT (NICE, 2011).

There are many talking therapies offered that you may have the opportunity to observe and learn about, including:

- *cognitive behavioural therapy (CBT)*: a talking therapy that helps people manage their problems by changing the way they think and behave

- *guided self-help*: service users work through a self-help workbook or computer course with the support of a therapist
- *counselling*: a talking therapy where a trained therapist listens to the service user and supports them to find ways to deal with emotional issues
- *interpersonal therapy*: a talking therapy that supports people with depression to identify and address problems in their relationships
- *behavioural activation*: a talking therapy that helps service users with depression to take simple, practical steps towards enjoying life again through increased motivation and problem-solving skills
- *eye movement desensitisation and reprocessing*: this therapy helps the brain reprocess memories of a traumatic event and has been developed to support service users with post-traumatic stress disorder (PTSD)
- *mindfulness-based cognitive therapy*: this therapy supports the service user to focus on their thoughts and feelings as they happen, combining mindfulness activities like meditation with cognitive therapy

Service users are generally seen in one-to-one or peer group sessions, focusing on a specific type of talking therapy suitable for their condition. If you have a placement with the IAPT service, you will observe the different dynamics and treatment styles, including one-to-one and group therapy. Service users are often given activities, such as CBT worksheets and mindfulness techniques, to continue at home between sessions.

Medication

Medication is often prescribed by GPs and psychiatrists to service users whose condition would benefit from pharmacological intervention. You may also see that an independent nurse prescriber prescribes medication for a particular service user group, within a defined remit.

Within any MH placement, you will be provided with an opportunity to explore and learn about the following in relation to medication management:

- the typical medications prescribed within that setting
- the desired benefits of prescribing these
- the potential side effects – physical and MH-related
- any contraindications related to physical health conditions and/or medications for physical conditions
- the advice given to service users about their medication

We will now explore some common MH medications in the next activity.

Activity 5.4   Critical thinking

Some of the commonly prescribed MH medications are listed below. Explore the literature and *British National Formulary Online* (https://about.medicinescomplete.

(Continued)

(Continued)

com/, accessed 25 May 2021) to identify the accepted reasons for prescribing these in an MH setting, their contraindications and their commonly experienced side effects:

- sertraline
- lorazepam
- risperidone
- lithium carbonate

An outline answer is given at the end of the chapter.

Alcohol detoxification services

Some services, such as community drug and alcohol services and alcohol detoxification units, offer inpatient and outpatient substance and alcohol detoxification. Here you will have the opportunity to undertake physical examination and observations before and during the service user's detox and observe for signs of withdrawal. Learning how to undertake a physical examination and observations are useful skills transferable to other settings. Service users may be admitted with acute withdrawal symptoms or with other physical health issues and then develop acute withdrawal whilst an inpatient. We will now explore this using a case study.

Case study: Paul

Paul is admitted for surgery for a fractured lower leg following an accident at work. While waiting on the ward for surgery, you notice that he is exhibiting signs of alcohol withdrawal. This may include sleep disturbances, anxiety, shaking, sweating and nausea.

How would you approach Paul to discuss this with him? You can review your thoughts on this in relation to the following section.

Supporting service users with alcohol withdrawal symptoms

When caring for service users such as Paul with potential acute alcohol withdrawal, it is important to utilise a nationally recognised alcohol screening tool. There are a number of these available, including Alcohol Use Disorders Identification Test for Consumption (AUDIT-C) and the Fast Alcohol Screening Tool (FAST) (PHE, 2020). As well as recognising and treating the clinical signs of alcohol misuse, it is important to offer referral to specialist alcohol services.

Structured brief advice should also be given to Paul or service users drinking hazardous or harmful amounts of alcohol using a recognised evidence-based resource that is based on the FRAMES principles (NICE, 2018a), which has the following steps:

- *Feedback*: on the service user's risk of having alcohol problems
- *Responsibility*: change is the persons' responsibility
- *Advice*: provision of clear advice
- *Menu*: options for change
- *Empathy*: reflective and understanding
- *Self-efficacy*: optimism about the service user's ability to change

Other treatments you may observe within mental health

Some specialist services offer alternative treatments, such as electroconvulsive therapy and neurosurgery, for severe and long-lasting MH conditions. If the service you are working within offers these, it is a useful learning opportunity to explore:

- the inclusion criteria for these treatments
- any contraindications
- the research/evidence base
- the service user information and consent process

Multidisciplinary working

Like all healthcare services, MH care cannot work in isolation, and therefore strong links with partner agencies are vital to ensure coordinated MH care for service users. We will start exploring this with the following activity.

Activity 5.5   Critical thinking

Similarly to all healthcare settings, there is cross-collaboration with other health professionals. Try to list all the different partner agencies that MH professionals need to work with to care for service users within MH.

An outline answer is given at the end of the chapter.

Partner agencies within MH

The agencies and roles with which MH services interact can broadly be separated into the following categories:

- other health services (primary, acute, physical healthcare, supportive therapies)
- social care
- voluntary organisations

MH services are separated into different tiers, and service users can move between tiers as their condition improves or deteriorates.

- *Tier 1*: refers to primary care offered by the service user's GP; this may be supportive consultations and/or prescription medications
- *Tier 2*: refers to generic community MH services, including IAPT
- *Tier 3*: refers to specialist treatments offered within the community setting
- *Tier 4*: are low-security inpatient MH services
- *Tiers 5 and 6*: are medium- and high-security inpatient MH services, typically for service users considered to pose a risk to others

It is important to note that a different tier system is used within Children and Adolescent Mental Health Services.

Caring for service users within each of the above tiers varies due to the number of complex MH issues service users can present with. As an NA student you may experience a range of emotions related to the above types of care. You may find this confusing, and very different to other areas of care. You may feel anxious or unsure about caring for service users in areas known as 'secure' areas, and areas being locked or having locked areas may cause you some questions. You may also be aware of service users who have current or previous convictions within 'forensic settings' and face some confusion about their care. These are complex issues and should be discussed with your PS and PA as you commence your placement.

Safeguarding in mental health

When talking about social care services, many people automatically think of safeguarding concerns. However, social care services bring a plethora of other support that service users can access. Many social care services work closely with community-based MH services, in particular, in order to provide holistic and effective multiagency support in the service user's home or community setting. You will learn how both services interact, their referral criteria and joint care planning for service users and families.

Case study: Prishna

You are observing a one-to-one session with Prishna, who is a service user with anxiety and depression. You are seeing her within an assessment unit. Prishna discloses to you that she is experiencing physical domestic abuse. You are already aware that Prishna lives with her husband and two young children.

Safeguarding 'is everybody's business' (HM Government, 2018), so you will have the opportunity to understand from an MH and social care perspective what is considered a safeguarding concern and the statutory process that is followed to protect vulnerable adults and children. This is often not straightforward, and a holistic multiprofessional approach is needed to assess any risks fully. Within the course of providing treatment for MH conditions, service users such as Prishna may disclose information that raises a safeguarding concern; therefore, it is important to understand your role and responsibilities around safeguarding and the local policies and procedures. This is an important area of learning you should discuss with your PA or PS, and it will be useful for you in other areas of practice.

Voluntary organisations to support families

Many voluntary organisations provide support for service users with MH concerns and their families, from Age Concern to Meals on Wheels to carers' support groups. It is important to understand what is offered in your local area so that you can signpost service users to the appropriate support. It may be that these organisations offer a type of support that your service cannot provide. Visiting these agencies whilst working within any MH setting enables you to understand their inclusion criteria and share these with colleagues, service users and families. Simple steps such as a daily hot meal or access to peer support can significantly improve an individual's MH.

Capacity to consent and deprivation of liberty

All service users are deemed to have the capacity to consent to treatment unless proven otherwise by a qualified practitioner (Mental Capacity Act, 2005). A choice that is considered unwise by a health professional does not necessarily mean that the service user cannot make that choice.

MH settings provide you with the opportunity to learn how the capacity to consent to treatment is assessed and the legal framework within which this sits. You may encounter service users without the capacity to consent in the community setting and service users who are considered to have full capacity in a secure forensic setting. It is important to understand what that means in relation to your role and the care you provide.

By placing a service user in a secure inpatient facility or providing one-to-one observation in an acute hospital setting, you are depriving a service user of their liberty, regardless of the capacity to consent. It is important to understand what this means in terms of the legal framework, your role and how this differs depending on the service user's age and condition.

Understanding these aspects is an important transferable skill, as you may care for a service user in a primary care setting who is unable to consent due to their MH condition, or you may deprive a service user of their liberty by placing them under constant observation due to concerns that they pose a risk to themselves in an Emergency Department. A service user detained under the Mental Health Act (1983) has been admitted for assessment or treatment against their expressed will. They may lack capacity or present with a severe clinical risk. This is often referred to as being 'sectioned' and is a unique learning opportunity in an MH placement, and would require discussion and debriefing with your PA or PS.

The five principles of capacity assessment as defined within the Mental Capacity Act (2005) are:

- Principle 1: the presumption of capacity

Capacity should be assumed unless proved otherwise.

Do not assume someone is unable to make a decision based on their medical condition or disability.

- Principle 2: support the individual

A service user should be given all possible help before they are deemed unable to make their own decisions.

Make every effort to support a service user in making a specific decision for themselves if possible.

- Principle 3: unwise decision

A service user has the right to make a decision that you might disagree with or consider irrational or unwise.

This doesn't indicate a lack of capacity, but may reflect individual preferences or values.

The ability to make the decision is key; not the decision itself.

- Principle 4: best interests

Decisions made or action taken for or on behalf of a person who lacks mental capacity must be done in their best interests.

'Best interests': These include a person's welfare, social, emotional and psychological interests as well as their medical interests.

Consider the service user's current or previous wishes and their beliefs and values (although these are not, in and of themselves, decisive).

- Principle 5: least restrictive option

If you're deciding on behalf of a person lacking capacity, you must consider whether it's possible to delay until the person regains capacity.

If a decision is needed, consider if you can do so while interfering with the person's rights or freedoms as little as possible.

If a person is temporarily incapacitated and you can defer the decision until they regain capacity, do so.

If this isn't possible, decide the person's best interests. The least restrictive option must be considered wherever possible.

Chapter summary

This chapter supports NA students to become aware of different types of care delivered within an MH setting. A significant difference between acute (physical) hospital care and MH care is an increased awareness of communication, enhanced safeguarding and capacity. Often service users with severe and enduring MH conditions may have fluctuating degrees of wellness, and it is essential to assess regularly whether the information given or new ideas are clearly understood. Skills such as OARS (open-ended questions, affirmations, reflections and summarising) assist in assuring information is being received or allows nurses to rephrase sentences for greater clarity. These concepts have been explored in this chapter.

The majority of care within MH is provided within the community setting, and this could be in specialist clinics or GP surgeries. This reduces the stigma for those receiving care, and integrates physical health with MH care needs. Medication is often used alongside other forms of therapy, including structured 'talking therapies', as explored. Individuals with MH conditions can also move between areas of care ranging from the GP surgery to forensic units, in the same way adults with physical care needs can require care from the GP, from the intensive care unit and from many services in between.

Activities: brief outline answers

Activity 5.2 Reflection

Your personal reflections on this will be different. This one is from a Year 1 student:

I observed a clinician giving a patient a distressing diagnosis with a poor prognosis in the open ward setting. The service user was understandably distressed by this news and appeared visibly shocked. There are many ways I feel that this situation could have been improved for the benefit of the service user. For example, I believe the service user would have felt better supported had there been a relative or staff present to support them whilst receiving this news. The fundamental principles I believe the service user would have wanted are empathy alongside honesty, the opportunity to ask a question and make choices about their care and time to process and understand the information being shared with them. It is important to support service users to receive information at their own pace and understanding and ensure they have the opportunity to ask further questions later. It is vital to actively listen to the service user's concerns and questions, as this will enable you to identify their understanding of the information shared. The use of rephrasing and paraphrasing their concerns allows me to show I am listening and keeps a person-centred approach. There are many ways I can support a service user who has recently received bad news, including expressing empathy, understanding, listening, supporting and empowering them to take an active role in their future care.

Tiana, Year 1 NA student

Activity 5.3 Evidence-based practice

MH conditions that may be supported by talking therapies include:

- depression
- anxiety
- grief and complex grief
- panic attacks
- phobias
- obsessive-compulsive disorder (OCD)
- PTSD
- some eating disorders
- stress
- perinatal depression and anxiety

Activity 5.4 Critical thinking

Sertraline

- Reason for prescribing: depressive illness, OCD, panic disorder, PTSD, social anxiety disorder
- Side effects: very common – chest pain, depression, gastrointestinal disorder, increased risk of infection, neuromuscular dysfunction, vasodilation
- Contraindications: poorly controlled epilepsy; selective serotonin reuptake inhibitors (SSRIs) should not be used if the service user enters a manic phase

Lorazepam

- Reason for prescribing: short-term anxiety, short-term use in insomnia associated with anxiety, panic attacks
- Side effects: decreased alertness; anxiety; ataxia (more common in elderly); confusion (more common in elderly); depression; dizziness; drowsiness; dysarthria; fatigue; gastrointestinal disorder; headache; hypotension; altered mood; muscle weakness; nausea; respiratory depression (particularly with a high dose and intravenous use – facilities for its treatment are essential); sleep disorders; suicidal ideation; tremor; vertigo; vision disorders; withdrawal syndrome
- Contraindications: acute pulmonary insufficiency; marked neuromuscular respiratory weakness; not for use alone to treat chronic psychosis (in adults); not for use alone to treat depression (or anxiety associated with depression) (in adults); obsessional states; phobic states; sleep apnoea syndrome; unstable myasthenia gravis; central nervous system depression; compromised airway; respiratory depression.

Risperidone

- Reason for prescribing: schizophrenia, acute and chronic psychosis, mania, short-term treatment (up to 6 weeks) of persistent aggression in service users with moderate to severe Alzheimer's dementia unresponsive to non-pharmacological interventions and when there is a risk of harm to self or others

- Side effects: agitation; amenorrhoea; arrhythmias; constipation; dizziness; drowsiness; dry mouth; erectile dysfunction; galactorrhoea; gynaecomastia; hyperprolactinaemia; hypotension (dose-related); insomnia; leucopenia; movement disorders; neutropenia; parkinsonism; QT interval prolongation; rash; seizure; tremor; urinary retention; vomiting; weight increase
- Contraindications: intramuscular use not to be used in children

Lithium carbonate

- Reason for prescribing: treatment and prophylaxis of mania, bipolar disorder, recurrent depression and aggressive or self-harming behaviour
- Side effects: abdominal discomfort; alopecia; angioedema; decreased appetite; arrhythmias; atrioventricular block; cardiomyopathy; cerebellar syndrome; circulatory collapse; coma; delirium; diarrhoea; dizziness; dry mouth; electrolyte imbalance; encephalopathy; folliculitis; gastritis; goitre; hyperglycaemia; hyperparathyroidism; hypersalivation; hypotension; hypothyroidism; idiopathic intracranial hypertension; leucocytosis; memory loss; movement disorders; muscle weakness; myasthenia gravis; nausea; neoplasms; nystagmus; peripheral neuropathy; peripheral oedema; polyuria; QT interval prolongation; abnormal reflexes; renal disorders; renal impairment; rhabdomyolysis; seizure; sexual dysfunction; skin reactions; skin ulcer; speech impairment; altered taste; thyrotoxicosis; tremor; vertigo; vision disorders; vomiting; increased weight
- Contraindications: Addison's disease; cardiac disease associated with rhythm disorder; cardiac insufficiency; dehydration; family history of Brugada syndrome; low-sodium diets; a personal history of Brugada syndrome; untreated hypothyroidism

Activity 5.5 Critical thinking

Partner agencies that MH professionals need to work with in order to care for service users within MH include:

- social care
- general practitioners
- health visitors and school nurses
- acute physical health services, including Accident and Emergency departments
- chronic pain services
- charities and voluntary organisations
- maternity services
- prisons
- Police
- occupational health
- occupational therapists
- universities and research units
- public health teams

Annotated further reading

NICE (2016) *Transition Between Inpatient Mental Health Settings and Community or Care Home Setting.* Available at: www.nice.org.uk/guidance/ng53/resources/transition-between-inservice-user-mental-health-settings-and-community-or-care-home-settings-pdf-1837511615941 (accessed 16 June 2021).

This guidance sets out the steps needed for the safe transition of service users between different services.

PHE (2018) *Health Matters: Reducing Health Inequalities in Mental Illness.* Available at: www.gov.uk/government/publications/health-matters-reducing-health-inequalities-in-mental-illness/health-matters-reducing-health-inequalities-in-mental-illness (accessed 16 June 2021).

This report explores the inequalities in heathcare faced by those with mental illness.

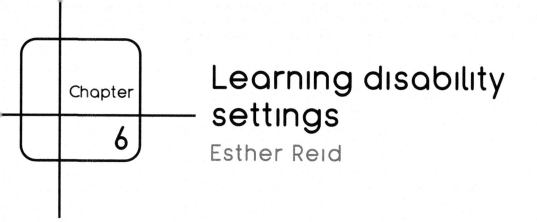

Learning disability settings

Esther Reid

(Continued)

6.4 understand the principles and processes involved in supporting people and families with a range of care needs to maintain optimal independence and avoid unnecessary interventions and disruptions to their lives.

6.5 identify when people need help to facilitate equitable access to care, support and escalate concerns appropriately.

Chapter aims

After reading this chapter, you will be able to:

- understand the complexities of providing care to people with learning disabilities.
- identify learning opportunities within a multidisciplinary team (MDT) in a learning disability setting.
- describe the transferable skills relevant to the context of your own work environment that you will gain from completing a learning disability placement.
- develop communication strategies that can be used when working with people with learning disabilities in any setting.
- demonstrate awareness of the barriers that people with learning disabilities face when accessing healthcare.

Introduction

This chapter will help you, as a Nursing Associate (NA) student, prepare for your practice placements in learning disability settings and will enable you to understand how the skills picked up in learning disability areas will enhance your practice in other settings. The chapter will consider the rationale for undertaking a learning disability placement and will explore strategies you can adopt to help you prepare for such placements. It will also explore the range of learning opportunities that may be available in these areas so that you can undertake relevant preparation. It is recognised that some NA students will have limited experience of working with people with learning disabilities, and may therefore feel apprehensive about their placement, so this chapter will cover some introductory information relating to learning disabilities, which can be read alongside the learning undertaken during your programme modules. The chapter will focus on communication skills and developing knowledge in relation to access to healthcare and reasonable adjustments which will be important areas of learning during the placement experience.

Not all NA students will undertake a placement experience in a specific learning disability team or setting, but you may have the opportunity to care for patients with learning disabilities in other settings and you will gain valuable learning from these experiences. Other opportunities include engaging with a patient's relative who has a learning disability. Whilst these engagements are not planned placements, it is important that you recognise them as an opportunity to enhance your understanding of learning disabilities. This chapter will enable you to feel more prepared for these opportunistic experiences.

Why have a learning disability placement?

Why is it so important that healthcare staff from all areas of nursing have the skills necessary to care for people with learning disabilities? The answer is straightforward. People with learning disabilities may, in the same way as any other member of the population, require medical intervention at various times throughout their life. This can be from attending a GP surgery for a blood test, being admitted on to a surgical ward for a hip replacement or being admitted to an acute medical area to treat an infection. You would be right to assume that people with learning disabilities should receive the same care as somebody without a learning disability when they are admitted to hospital. Sadly, this is not always the case.

People with learning disabilities are more likely to experience physical and mental health problems than people without a learning disability. It is important to acknowledge that the life expectancy of people with learning disabilities is lower than of the general population: 17 years shorter for women with learning disabilities and 14 years shorter for men with learning disabilities (NHS Digital, 2020). The Confidential Inquiry into Premature Deaths of People with Learning Disabilities (Heslop et al., 2013) found that 38% of people with a learning disability died from a cause that could have been avoided by the provision of good-quality healthcare.

Student tip 6.1

Following my learning disability placement I felt more confident in supporting people with learning disabilities when they were admitted on to my ward area. I found it helpful to share my learning with other members of the team so that we could ensure consistency in our approach and it helped with building the confidence of other staff.

Aliyah, Year 2 NA student

Before we move on to considering learning disability placements, it is useful to reflect on your understanding of learning disabilities.

Activity 6.1   Critical thinking

What does the term 'learning disability' mean to you? What do you consider to be some of the common conditions associated with learning disabilities?

As this is a personal activity, there is no outline answer at the end of the chapter.

Completing Activity 6.1 will have allowed you to consider your own understanding of learning disabilities and you may have identified what you believe to be common associated conditions. We will now explore the most common definition of learning disabilities and identify some commonly associated conditions for you to compare your answers to.

Learning disability and commonly associated conditions

The most well-known definition of learning disability, as explained by the Department of Health (2001) in their white paper *Valuing People*, is as follows:

- a significantly reduced ability to understand new or complex information
- a reduced ability to learn new skills and cope independently
- must have started before adulthood with a long-lasting effect on development

A learning disability happens when a person's brain development is affected before they are born, during birth or early in their childhood. Learning disability can be caused by the mother becoming ill during pregnancy, problems during birth that prevent enough oxygen reaching the brain, illness or injury in early childhood or the baby inheriting certain genes that make a learning disability more likely. In some cases, there is no known cause for a learning disability.

Along with the above definition, learning disabilities can be described in terms of severity as follows:

- mild – will need very little support and can often go undiagnosed
- moderate – will be able to communicate most needs but may require some support in everyday tasks
- severe – some communication skills and will need support with most everyday tasks
- profound and multiple – may have multiple disabilities and need the highest level of support

There are a number of conditions associated with learning disability that you will encounter during your placement experience. This may include the following:

- Down's syndrome – genetic condition caused by the presence of an extra chromosome 21
- Edward's syndrome – a rare but serious genetic condition caused by the presence of a third copy of all or part of chromosome 18
- Fragile X syndrome – a genetic condition that can affect both males and females, although males are more severely affected
- Cerebral palsy – a physical condition that affects movement, posture and coordination, usually caused by an injury to the brain before, during or shortly after birth

- Autism – autism refers to a broad range of conditions and is not a learning disability, although approximately half of autistic people may also have a learning disability

It is important to acknowledge that the above is not an exhaustive list of associated conditions, but it is included to give you an idea of the conditions you may encounter as part of your placement experience. If your placement area is related to some specific conditions, it will be helpful to read further around those. You will discover that each condition impacts on individuals in different ways. This will allow you to appreciate the importance of researching conditions so that the care you provide can be adapted in order to meet the specific needs of the person.

Learning from learning disability settings

Having considered what a learning disability is and some of the common associated conditions, this section will explore learning from learning disability settings and consider the transferable skills that can be developed as part of this experience.

Activity 6.2 Evidence-based practice and research

What is your understanding of the services available that specifically support people with learning disabilities? Where have you searched for information when you have had to support a person with a learning disability?

As this is a personal activity, there is no outline answer at the end of the chapter.

Organisations that support people with learning disabilities

Now that you have considered your understanding of the services available to people with learning disabilities, this section will identify the types of organisations and settings that work to support people with learning disabilities in all aspects of life. It is important to remember that placements will vary depending on where in the country you are located. You will have the opportunity to complete these practice learning experiences in settings that reflect the diversity of the services that may be accessed by people with a learning disability. This may include the following:

- Community learning disability teams – these teams provide specialist healthcare to adults with learning disabilities who have needs that cannot be met by mainstream services alone. Professionals working within these teams help to ensure that people with learning disabilities receive the same care and treatment as the general population. In order to achieve this, they undertake assessments and produce evidence-based care plans in consultation with the individual and those supporting them on a day-to-day basis.

- Nursing and residential homes – these services provide high-quality care which is personalised to the individual's needs. People with a learning disability living within these settings will be encouraged to take part in everyday activities with support provided which aims to give people as much control as possible over their life.
- Supported living services – these services work together with other organisations, social and private landlords in order to find accommodation that meets the need of the individual. These services can also provide personal support to people that ranges from a couple of hours a week to 24 hours a day, 7 days a week.
- Short-break respite services – these services are designed for people with a learning disability and their families in order to give them a change from their usual routine. They also enable parents and carers to have a break from their carer role. These services may support people in the family home or may be offered in short-break facilities.

You may also have the opportunity to work within educational settings, employment services, forensic services, prisons and palliative care services. Learning disability placements may be undertaken in community settings within the National Health Service, local authority, independent or voluntary organisations. In the same way as with other placements, you may have the opportunity to access a range of experiences across a 24-hour period by undertaking early, late and night shifts.

There are a number of key organisations that support people with a learning disability and their family. The following list is not exhaustive of the services that offer support, but has been included as a starting point for you to be able to seek further information depending on where you are allocated for your placement. The list below may also be useful if you require further advice in relation to your own work setting.

- Mencap: www.mencap.org.uk/
- National Autistic Society: www.autism.org.uk/
- British Institute of Learning Disabilities: www.bild.org.uk/
- Down's Syndrome Association: www.downs-syndrome.org.uk/
- Foundation for People with Learning Disabilities: www.learningdisabilities.org.uk/
- Scope www.scope.org.uk/

The multidisciplinary team working with people with a learning disability

An MDT approach when supporting people with a learning disability is vital in order to increase opportunity for people. During your placement in a learning disability setting you will likely have the opportunity to work with various professionals and this will add depth to your learning experience. It is possible that you may support a service user to attend a GP appointment, observe a hydrotherapy session with a physiotherapist or observe the ways in which a speech and language therapist supports people with a learning disability to communicate. Whatever the experience you encounter, it is important to recognise how these members of the MDT improve the lives of people with a learning disability. The MDT in this context includes:

- doctor (general practitioner (GP), psychiatrist)
- nurse (community learning disability nurse, hospital liaison nurse, specialist nurse, NA, student nurse, student NA)
- physiotherapist
- occupational therapist
- social worker
- dietician
- speech and language therapist
- psychologist

Learning opportunities in learning disability settings

Prior to commencing your placement in a learning disability setting, it is important to consider the learning opportunities available to you and how you can develop transferable skills that will benefit you in your future role. There are a number of components that can be considered as relevant in relation to education for all healthcare students in the area of learning disability. Examples of this learning include:

- *Communication* – you will encounter people who have significant communication impairments. This will include people with limited or no verbal communication, those who use communication aids and others who are reliant on body language, gestures and facial expressions. Communication strategies will be covered later in this chapter.
- *Attitudes towards people with learning disabilities* – people with learning disabilities often face negative attitudes and, in the context of healthcare, this can have a detrimental effect on the outcomes for these people. Gaining experience from a learning disability placement can help to build confidence, which in turn can improve attitudes.
- *Reasonable adjustments* (Equality Act 2010) – there is much guidance available on making reasonable adjustments within healthcare for people with learning disabilities. This will be covered in more detail later in this chapter.
- *Health needs of people with learning disabilities* – this may include supporting people with learning disabilities to attend appointments, for example, the dentist or their GP. You may also have the opportunity to familiarise yourself with commonly used documentation which assists people with learning disabilities when they have their health needs met, such as hospital passports (these are explained later in this chapter).
- *Handover* – handovers that you observe in learning disability settings may be different to those that you have observed in other areas due to the nature of care that is provided in these settings. Involvement in these handovers is really

important to enable you to develop your understanding of people with learning disabilities.

- *Awareness of diagnostic overshadowing* – diagnostic overshadowing occurs when the symptoms of physical ill health are considered inherent to a person's learning disability or are incorrectly attributed to a person's behavioural issues. An example of this would be where a person with a learning disability starts to display self-injurious behaviour by hitting their chest repeatedly. It could be that the person is experiencing chest pain and this is their way of expressing the pain. However, if the person is known to have challenging behaviour, the chest pain could be missed as the behaviour is wrongly attributed to their behavioural issue.
- *Capacity, consent and best interests* – you may have already gained some experience on matters of capacity and consent in other placement areas, but this is managed very differently for people with learning disabilities and often staff have to adopt principles of best interests.

Other learning opportunities that are specific to certain areas may include the following:

- *Nutrition and hydration* – this may include supporting service users with nutrition and hydration orally or via alternative routes such as percutaneous endoscopic gastrostomy or nasogastric tubes.
- *Administration of medication under supervision* – it is particularly important to develop knowledge of medication contraindications and how these may be evident in someone with a learning disability. They may not be able to communicate side effects verbally so you must be able to look out for other signs that they are feeling unwell.
- *Moving and handling* – some people with a learning disability will have an associated physical disability resulting in reduced mobility. This may result in them needing physical assistance. If you are allocated to a placement area that supports people in this way, you will be able to develop your skill in using hoists and other pieces of equipment for moving and handling.
- *Challenging behaviour* – it is important to be aware that people with a learning disability are more likely to show challenging behaviour. This can be due to a difficulty with communication, meaning that people with a learning disability display challenging behaviours in order to express frustration. Challenging behaviour can also be a sign that someone is in pain or discomfort. Whilst it would be difficult to develop competence in working with people who show challenging behaviours during a short placement experience, you should seek opportunity to improve your understanding in this area in order to improve the way you support people.

The above lists are not exhaustive and there will be many other learning opportunities specific to the setting you are allocated to. The important thing is to be open-minded about your learning and think carefully about how you can apply your learning to your permanent setting.

Effective communication skills for supporting people with learning disabilities

The next section will explore communication methods that can be used when supporting people with learning disabilities. These skills can be further developed during your placement. Before we explore some specific communication strategies, it will be useful to consider your knowledge so far in this area.

Activity 6.3   Reflection

Think of a patient you have supported who had either a learning disability or a communication impairment. How did you feel prior to interacting with them? Were there any strategies you adopted in order to communicate effectively?

An outline answer is given at the end of the chapter.

When working with people with learning disabilities, it is important that staff recognise the need to adapt their communication methods in order to be understood by people who have a communication impairment. This is why communication will be a key area of learning during this placement and you should make the most of this opportunity to develop your skills. People with a learning disability do not always have a level of understanding that enables them to understand the spoken and written word, therefore healthcare professionals must enhance their communication through additional verbal and non-verbal communication skills. We will now consider some of these skills and their importance in communication within this context. The following tips may be a useful starting point:

- Non-verbal communication:
  - eye contact
  - gestures
  - body language
  - use of real objects as a communication aid
  - use of photos, pictures and symbols for key words
- Careful use of verbal communication:
  - Always speak to the person first and not to the people supporting them.
  - Speak clearly and not too fast.
  - Avoid jargon, abbreviations and metaphors.
  - Use concrete terms rather than figurative language and avoid abstracts.
  - Use straightforward language and simply constructed sentences.
  - Ask open questions.

- o Start your conversation by asking some questions you know the person can answer to reduce anxiety and build confidence.
- o Allow more time for the person to think and construct their answer.
- o Ask questions to clarify that the person has understood what you have said and check with the person that you have understood what they are saying.

Activity 6.4   Communication skills

Reflect on your own level of skill for each of the communication strategies listed above. How many of these have you used? Are there any that you haven't tried but think would be useful in your work area when communicating with people with learning disabilities?

As this is a personal activity, there is no outline answer at the end of the chapter.

Developing effective communication skills

You may have reflected on the above activity and come to the conclusion that you have a lot of development to do in terms of your communication skills, particularly in your use of language, and be wondering how your learning disability placement will help you. One of the main ways that you will develop effective communication skills is by working alongside people who have a learning disability and the people who know them well. It is important that you observe the skills that others around you adopt when interacting with service users. It is also important that you are aware of the differing communication methods that people with learning disabilities may use. This can range from something as simple as a gesture through to visual aids or specialist technology. We all use gestures, body language and facial expressions in our day-to-day communication but these skills are all the more important when communicating with people with learning disabilities.

Student tip 6.2

I felt really nervous prior to starting my learning disability placement because I was worried I wouldn't understand what the service users were saying to me. I didn't want to upset anyone by saying the wrong thing. Whilst I found some service users difficult to understand initially, as I spent more time with them, I found I was able to 'tune in' to their speech. I would advise any other student feeling the same way as I did to just spend as much time with the service users as possible and be patient with yourself.

Raymond, Year 2 NA student

Case study: Francesca

Francesca is 35 years old and has cerebral palsy and a learning disability. She is admitted to the medical ward where you work as an NA student, as she has developed pneumonia. Her cerebral palsy means that she needs full support in all aspects of care and she is unable to communicate verbally. She relies on visual communication boards and those who know her well in order to make her needs known. She usually lives at home with her parents and they try to spend as much time as possible with her on the ward.

You are working a night shift and Francesca's parents have gone home in order to get some rest. Francesca has been sleeping well during her time in hospital but on this occasion she wakes in the early hours of the morning and starts showing signs of distress. The nurse in charge asks you to go and support her. You are unsure why she is upset and you know that the team have been relying on Francesca's parents being present in order to communicate with her. You find a communication book on the chair next to her bed containing a series of pages with symbols and photographs.

Francesca's situation is an example of one you could find yourself in on a shift. Quite often there is a reliance on family members or care staff remaining with the person throughout their stay in hospital, but this is not always sustainable for long periods of time. Activity 6.5 asks you to explore your options in this situation and identify some strategies which you could adopt to support Francesca.

Activity 6.5   Critical thinking

Having read the case study about Francesca, reflect on the following questions:

- What would you do in this situation?
- What transferable skills from a learning disability placement could help you support Francesca?

An outline answer is given at the end of the chapter.

Student tip 6.3

I had limited experience of supporting people with learning disabilities prior to studying the NA programme. I found that reading information on common conditions associated with learning disabilities and watching videos that shared examples on how people with learning disabilities communicate helped me to know what to expect. I'm glad I did this before my placement.

Luis, Year 1 NA student

Access to healthcare and reasonable adjustments

It is important to develop awareness of the barriers that exist which prevent people with a learning disability from accessing good-quality healthcare, in order to ensure that you work to improve access for these people. It is therefore vital that you are aware how to make reasonable adjustments for people with learning disabilities. Reasonable adjustments are a legal requirement under the Equality Act (2010) whereby public sector organisations must make changes in their provision to ensure that services are accessible to disabled people.

There are a number of barriers that stop people with a learning disability from receiving good-quality healthcare and you may see these for yourself during your placement. It is important that you know what to look out for so that you can acknowledge a particular issue as a barrier and know how to work to prevent it in future. Some of the barriers include:

- difficulty in attending appointments due to a lack of accessible transport
- staff having little or no understanding about learning disability and how this affects individuals
- staff feeling anxious or lacking confidence when supporting people with a learning disability
- lack of joint working between different care providers who work to support a person with a learning disability
- failure to recognise that a person with a learning disability is actually unwell. This can be particularly difficult if the person does not display symptoms in a way that would be expected
- failure to correctly diagnose a condition. As mentioned earlier in the chapter, diagnostic overshadowing can be a particular issue in achieving an accurate diagnosis
- inadequate follow-up care

A number of reasonable adjustments can be made to improve the experiences people with a learning disability have when accessing mainstream healthcare. Hospital passports are a key development in improving these experiences; they should be with the person and taken to all different locations of care with them. These documents provide important information about a person with a learning disability, including personal details, medication and pre-existing health conditions. They also include details about a person's communication and their likes and dislikes. Hospital passports should be with the person at each stage of their healthcare, but they are not always used appropriately or effectively. It is important that you take the time during your learning disability placement to familiarise yourself with them. This will help you in your future practice to use them effectively.

Public Health England (2018) have shared good practice advice in making reasonable adjustments for people with learning disabilities. Some examples of reasonable adjustments that you may observe and could consider in your own practice are as follows:

- utilising the skills and knowledge of staff who regularly support the person
- improving appointments by allowing more time for tasks and reducing long periods of waiting time
- creating positive environments that do not increase anxiety by taking into account noise levels, lighting and equipment that may be on show and could cause unnecessary distress
- minimising the number of different people who need to assess and treat the person
- effective use of accessible information

Accessible information for people with learning disabilities

This final section will consider the ways in which we present information to people with a learning disability when, for example, we need to perform a procedure such as taking a blood sample or dressing a wound. Before the information is shared, it is important to consider what you already do to explain relevant information to people with learning disabilities.

Activity 6.6   Reflection

Consider the clinical skills and procedures that are frequently carried out within your work area and write these down. Reflect on the ways in which information about these procedures is shared with patients; for example patient information leaflets, posters, etc. Now consider how this information is shared with people who have learning disabilities. How easy is it to understand the medical terminology associated with the skills/procedure? Do you have access to accessible information? How can you help a patient's understanding if they are unable to read or can only communicate non-verbally?

This may also be something you want to discuss with staff in your area if you think you should be doing more to make information more accessible for people.

An outline answer is given at the end of the chapter.

Now that you have reflected on the methods you already use to explain information to people who may not be able to read standard information leaflets, we will consider why accessible information for people with learning disabilities is so vital and how you can improve your skill in effectively utilising accessible information. Your work area may be well resourced with leaflets written in an accessible format, but how can you use them in your practice?

Providing people who have a learning disability with accessible information can be helpful in engaging them with their health and the care they receive, which in turn can help to reduce their anxieties and the health inequalities identified earlier. A benefit of accessible information is that, in a number of cases, it can allow a person to review the information independently, but it is important to remember that it should not replace conversation and some people will still need support to read and understand the document. This is another opportunity for learning during your learning disability placement. In Activity 6.6 you may have reflected on an experience where either you did not have accessible information to share with a patient, or you may have had a leaflet but still found that it did not work or know how to use it to help the person understand. Your skill development during your learning disability placement, the information shared in this chapter in relation to communication and your awareness of your workplace and how accessible information could be helpful will enable you to improve your practice.

Case study: Xavier

Xavier is 42 years old and has Down's syndrome and a moderate learning disability. He has recently been suffering from hearing loss as a result of a build-up of earwax. Xavier has been seen by his GP several times but has been unable to tolerate the procedure to clear the wax from his ears. Xavier has been seen regularly by a speech and language therapist in order to develop alternative methods of communication whilst he is unable to hear, but this is not considered to be a long-term solution. It was therefore recommended that Xavier be admitted to hospital in order for the earwax to be removed under general anaesthetic.

You are working on the surgical ward where Xavier is due to be admitted and you have been asked to prepare for Xavier's admission to hospital.

Activity 6.7   Critical thinking

Make some notes as to what you could do in order to prepare for Xavier's admission to hospital. What could you offer to Xavier to prepare him for his admission and what skills would you need to consider using to support him during his time on your ward?

An outline answer is given at the end of the chapter.

Chapter summary

This chapter has introduced you to the learning you can expect from a learning disability placement. It is important to recognise the value of having a learning disability placement in order to improve your level of skill and develop your understanding of learning disabilities, which will improve the experience these people have when accessing healthcare.

Introductory information relating to learning disabilities and common associated conditions has been provided in order to enable you to understand what it means to have a learning disability. Specific transferable skills that you will develop during your placement have been explored, with a focus on communication skills, which will allow you to prepare for your placement and manage your expectations. The chapter finished by exploring access to healthcare and developing understanding of reasonable adjustments that can be further explored during your placement.

It is important to understand that this is a huge area of learning and whilst this chapter has covered some important aspects, wider reading is essential. It is hoped that the learning from reading this chapter along with your modules of study will assist you with the necessary preparation prior to commencing a learning disability placement, which in turn will enable you to gain the most from this experience.

Activities: brief outline answers

Activity 6.3 Reflection

When considering this reflection, you may have identified feelings of uncertainty when considering how best to communicate. You may also have identified a feeling of nervousness that you would communicate in the wrong way and not be understood. These are very common feelings when faced with a situation that requires the use of unfamiliar methods of communication. Some of the strategies identified may have included observing the ways in which a family member or carer communicated with the person, being mindful of your positioning so that the person could observe your body language and making sure you used eye contact appropriately. You might also have considered your use of language and whether you used any pictures, symbols or objects to complement your verbal communication.

Activity 6.5 Critical thinking

When considering the case study about Francesca, you would need to apply the communication skills developed during your learning disability placement in order to find out why Francesca is distressed. As a starting point, you could ask one of your colleagues if they have observed how Francesca uses her communication book. In addition, you should look for a guide within her communication book which tells people how she uses the symbols and photographs to communicate. It would be worthwhile locating her hospital passport as this should include detail about her communication. You would need to ensure you allocate enough time to sit with her in order to work through her communication book. In this scenario, it is important not to make assumptions about why she might be distressed. There could be a number of factors causing her upset and you must be open-minded in order to interpret what she is actually expressing.

Activity 6.6 Reflection

You will hopefully have written a list of clinical skills and procedures that are frequently used within your work area. When reflecting on the ways in which information about these procedures is shared with patients, you may have identified that you mostly use verbal explanations and sometimes support them with patient information leaflets. When considering the medical terminology associated with the skill or procedure, you may have come to the conclusion that the terminology used is sometimes difficult to understand and that we often use it without considering alternative explanations. When reflecting on ways to help a patient's understanding if they are unable to read or can only communicate non-verbally, you may have considered the use of pictures and symbols within accessible information leaflets. You may also have reviewed the communication strategies identified in this chapter and decided that you could use signing, gestures or real objects to communicate.

Activity 6.7 Critical thinking

Your answer to this may have included the following:

- Contact Xavier in advance to offer a visit to the ward so that he can familiarise himself with the environment and meet the people who will be caring for him.
- Enquire if Xavier has a hospital passport and request to view this prior to his admission. Make sure the hospital passport is read by everyone who will be working with Xavier.
- Find out further information about the communication strategies he has been using so that these can be adopted during his admission, particularly before the procedure.
- Ensure he is allocated to an appropriate area on the ward, taking into account the level of noise, access to support and anything else that may cause Xavier distress during his admission.
- Consider the timing of his procedure and the time that he therefore is required to arrive at the hospital. It would be beneficial to reduce waiting time for Xavier in order to reduce his anxiety.

Annotated further reading

Emerson, E., Baines, S., Allerton, L. and Welsh, V. (2012) *Health Inequalities & People with Learning Disabilities in the UK: 2012*. London: Department of Health. Available at: www.researchgate.net/publication/275208195_Health_Inequalities_and_People_With_Learning_Disabilities_in_the_UK (accessed 28 February 2012).

This document summarises the health status of people with learning disabilities in the UK and explains the health inequalities they face.

Hamon, L. and Clift, J. (2011) *General Hospital Care for People with Learning Disabilities.* West Sussex: John Wiley.

This book is a resource for professionals working in a hospital setting who may come into contact with people with learning disabilities.

Hardy, S., Chaplin, E. and Woodward, P. (2016) *Supporting the Physical Health Needs of People with Learning Disabilities. A Handbook for Professionals, Support Staff and Families.* East Sussex: Pavilion Publishing and Media.

This book provides a practical guide to a range of physical illnesses and health needs experienced by people with a learning disability and details of how to support people with these conditions.

Mencap (2007) *Death by Indifference.* London: Mencap.

Mencap (2012) *Death by Indifference: 74 Deaths and Counting.* London: Mencap.

These Mencap documents both highlight the inequalities that people with a learning disability experience, by reporting on a number of deaths of people with learning disabilities, which have been deemed avoidable had they received appropriate healthcare.

Annotated useful websites

Easy Health – this website contains health leaflets written in an accessible format using pictures and simple text.

www.easyhealth.org.uk/

Foundation for People with Learning Disabilities – this website includes the latest learning disability-related news and information as well as providing a forum for people who have questions about supporting people with learning disabilities.

www.learningdisabilities.org.uk/

Mencap – The voice of learning disability. This page contains advice and useful information relating to learning disability and the support available:

www.mencap.org.uk/

National Institute for Health and Care Excellence – People with learning disabilities. This page includes guidance, advice, NICE pathways and quality standards:

www.nice.org.uk/guidance/population-groups/people-with-learning-disabilities

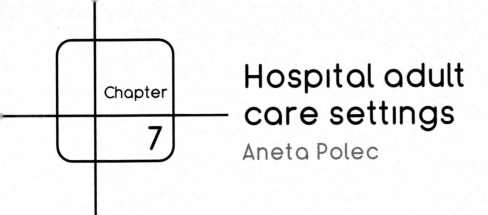

Chapter 7

Hospital adult care settings

Aneta Polec

Platform 6: Contributing to integrated care

At the point of registration, the nursing associate will be able to:

6.2   understand and explore the challenges of providing safe nursing care for people with complex co-morbidities and complex care needs.

6.3   demonstrate an understanding of the complexities of providing mental, cognitive, behavioural and physical care needs across a wide range of integrated care settings.

Chapter aims

By the end of this chapter you should be able to:

- demonstrate understanding of the main adult care settings in the hospital.
- identify learning opportunities available on medical and surgical wards.
- ascertain which proficiencies are likely to be achievable in each setting.
- identify potential multidisciplinary learning opportunities while undertaking placements in adult care settings.

Introduction

In Chapter 3 you explored how care can be delivered to patients in primary care settings. The current health policy of the UK Government aims to cut down on the number of hospital admissions by provision of appropriate services in the community (Smith et al., 2014). Nevertheless, patients will still require treatment in hospital for a variety of conditions that cannot be treated at home, or when they need to undergo a procedure or surgery. During your programme you may be allocated to a placement on a hospital ward, and this type of placement will provide the perfect opportunity for you to practise basic nursing skills and learn how to deliver holistic patient care. This chapter will cover the key concepts of patient care and learning opportunities in adult care such as medical or surgical ward settings. Interprofessional working and learning opportunities will also be explored.

An overview of adult care settings in a hospital

The reason for admission to hospital will vary from being referred by the GP, after presenting to the Accident and Emergency (A&E) department (see Chapter 8) following an accident and being brought in by ambulance, as well as due to the need for surgery.

Following initial triage in A&E, a patient will be admitted to one of the hospital wards, and subject to the reason for admission, this could be a surgical or medical ward. Depending on the hospital speciality, and whether it is a National Health Service (NHS) hospital or an independent one run by private companies or charities, surgical and medical wards are the two most common types of adult settings and these will be explored in detail in this chapter. In general, medical wards include settings such as acute assessment areas, frailty and elderly settings and specialist areas such gastroenterology, hepatobiliary, stroke, cardiology, respiratory and infectious diseases, whilst surgical areas include acute assessment, gynaecology, musculoskeletal and many others, including plastic surgery.

Preparing for placements in adult care settings

Activity 7.1 Evidence-based practice and research

Look at all areas within your local Trust and try to determine if they are broadly medicine or surgery. Try to come up with ideas on what you will be able to learn and observe if you were to have a placement in one or more of those areas.

An outline answer is given at the end of the chapter.

When thinking of learning opportunities on medical and surgical wards, you probably came up with simple nursing tasks like administration of medicines, attending to wounds and looking after the patient following surgery. This chapter will explore many more and hopefully provide you with ideas on what can be expected and how this experience could benefit your learning.

As mentioned in Chapter 1, it is important that you spend some time preparing for your placement regardless of where it is. The advantage of the hospital setting is that, once you have experienced a placement on the ward and get used to the shift patterns, daily routine, basic equipment and terms used by healthcare professionals, this is likely to be similar and comparable whichever other ward you are placed on in the future. This should help alleviate some of the anxieties you may have about attending a new placement area. It is still crucial, however, that you take your time to learn about the ward area before you commence. Refer back to Chapter 1 for detailed advice on how to prepare for a clinical placement.

Hospital ward organisation

This chapter will focus on medical and surgical wards separately and will discuss the unique learning opportunities as well as the members of the team you are likely to meet. Before that, let us look at some features which are common to the majority of adult hospital wards, regardless of their speciality.

Off-duty allocation

Off-duty, also called a roster or rota, is usually prepared months in advance, as it takes into consideration the ward demands, patient flow and staff annual leave. The off-duty can be kept on the ward in a hard-copy format while other departments may use an electronic version. There may be a separate roster for students or it may be incorporated into the staff roster.

Student tip 7.1

It is a good idea to find out where the off-duty is kept on the ward on your first day of placement and familiarise yourself with shifts scheduled for you for the forthcoming weeks so that you can be confident you know when to turn up. It helped me to find out who was the nominated person amongst the ward staff to deal with and modify the off-duty and I referred to this person only if I had specific requests or amendments.

Ade, Year 2 Nursing Associate (NA) student

Shift pattern

You will be informed about the shift pattern before you commence your placement or during induction. The majority of hospital wards nowadays implement 'long-day' and night shift patterns, while others will allow for 'half-day' shifts. It is recommended that when you are a student on the programme you work the majority of day shifts, as a lot of learning opportunities take place during the day. You may however be asked to work a few night shifts over the course of your programme (depending on the unit's needs and availability of practice supervisor (PS)) as they can provide you with valuable experiences. This will ensure you can support and take part in the 24-hour cycle of care. Please make sure you discuss this with your practice assessor (PA) or the manager.

Ward daily routine

The shift usually starts with the handover and allocation of staff to each bay/room of patients. Depending on the arrangement, a group handover can take place in the designated area or an individual handover at a patient's bedside. Regardless of whether you are provided with a printed handover or you are encouraged to make your own notes, make sure you dispose of the notes appropriately at the end of the shift in order to protect patient confidentiality (NMC, 2018d).

Many hospital wards have started implementing safety huddles throughout the day. Huddles are short meetings between professionals involved in patient care giving them a chance to discuss patients' needs, introduced as a safety measure to improve patient outcomes (Montague et al., 2019).

When on placement you are encouraged to work as part of the team. As mentioned in Chapter 1, you are encouraged to advocate for your role, and one way to achieve this could be by making sure that your name and the role of NA student are clearly identified on the daily team allocation board. You are likely to be allocated to work alongside a qualified member of staff or look after your own group of patients under supervision (depending on your year of study). Make sure that you negotiate your break times and be prepared to relieve other members of staff to allow for theirs.

Student tip 7.2

I soon developed the habit of clarifying before each placement started whether my status was supernumerary, or whether I would be counted among the staff numbers. This was important so that appropriate protected learning time could be allocated to promote my learning and progression. I also never assumed that I would be allocated to work alongside another member of staff under their direct supervision.

Mohammed, Year 2 NA student

After some time spent on the ward you may notice a pattern of how the day/night shift is run. The morning shift could start by providing patients with personal hygiene needs, followed by breakfast and the medication round. On the other hand the night shift could commence with the medication round followed by providing personal hygiene needs. Note that ward routines can be altered to ensure we are responsive to patients' needs and respect their choices and preferences as patients have the right to make decisions about their care (NMC, 2018d).

The daily routine can easily be disrupted by an emergency (like a cardiac arrest), outbreak of infectious disease which could require intra-hospital transfer of patients between the wards or a major incident having an impact on A&E and consequently on all of the wards in hospital. Therefore, you need to be prepared to work flexibly and understand that, while your development is very important, there may be times when unexpected pressures on staff and resources will affect your learning opportunities.

Activity 7.2   Critical thinking

We have already discussed how important it is to dispose of the nursing handover notes in order to avoid breaches in confidentiality. As a member of the team you will have access to other sensitive information regarding patients in your care, like their medical notes and test results. What is your legal and professional duty with regard to those? Can you think of any relevant documents that provide healthcare professionals with guidance in this area? Now look at your Practice Assessment Document (PAD) and identify those proficiencies focusing on documentation, handover and confidentiality.

An outline answer is given at the end of the chapter.

While on placement you are likely to be able to access patients' notes on the central database used by individual hospital. This means that you use the system both to input the data relevant to a patient's current admission and also to access past medical history (PMH) and personal identifiable information. It is crucial that you understand the principles of sharing confidential information regarding patients in your care and, if you are given a unique passcode to access those details, you should never share this with other members of staff.

Multidisciplinary working on adult hospital wards

You are likely to come across certain members of the team regardless of which hospital ward you are allocated to.

Cleaners, also called the domestic team, are responsible for maintaining cleanliness in the clinical area, including disposal of contaminated as well as non-hazardous waste.

There will nearly always be a ward clerk responsible for general administration of the ward. They may look after patients' records, answer the phone and greet patients, relatives and visitors as they come in.

Catering assistants will deal with patient food orders and preferences as well as delivery of meals at specific times during the day.

Porters are responsible for transfer of patients who require a trolley or a wheelchair as well as transport of blood samples and blood products. They also deal with linen, post, stores and equipment.

A ward manager will be responsible for the daily running of the ward and provision of services, allocation of staff, making sure the ward environment is risk-managed, just to name the few. This could be a senior member of nursing staff. They will work alongside a matron, who is responsible for overseeing a particular speciality or a suite of areas that work together and usually has a very high degree of specialist knowledge. Managers and matrons will work closely with bed managers and discharge coordinators who are responsible for placement of patients arriving at the hospital and facilitation of timely and safe discharges.

The clinical team on the ward comprises doctors with various levels of seniority, nurses (bands 5–7), healthcare support workers, NAs and students, all involved in direct patient care.

Wards are regularly visited by pharmacists, who are able to review patients' medication, advise on appropriate substitutions or medications requiring complex preparation as well as prepare the medications for patient discharge (to take home).

Volunteers are often seen supporting ward areas; their role may include providing patient comfort measures or organisation of the ward area.

Learning opportunities on hospital ward related to patient care

Irrespective of the speciality of the adult hospital setting you have been allocated to, you will notice there will usually be certain activities taking place regularly in those areas. Participation in these will help you achieve your objectives set at the beginning of each placement, as well as the proficiencies outlined in your PAD, such as the following.

Monitoring of vital signs

For some of you this will be a completely new skill to learn, while other students will be familiar with undertaking observations, as they will have learnt this in their place of work. Monitoring of vital signs is one of the most commonly performed monitorings of a patient in hospital. Vital signs are used to assess and evaluate a patient's progress and consist of checking respiratory rate, oxygen saturations, blood pressure, pulse rate, temperature and consciousness level (Peate, 2019). If you have never done this skill before, you will be given the chance to practise each vital sign under supervision before you are deemed competent to perform them independently.

Medication management

Adult care settings in hospital provide an excellent opportunity for students to develop knowledge, skills and competencies in the area of medicines administration. You will be given the chance to assess the patient prior to medication administration, prepare, administer and assess the efficacy of medications and document your actions. The majority of this will be done at the patient's bedside; however the preparation of medication can sometimes take place in the treatment room where the medication cupboard is located. Hospital wards are still using medication trolleys – a lockable trolley stocked with basic medications that can be taken around the ward. It is good practice to take note of the most commonly used medications, and then refer to a textbook in order to find out what they are used for, how they work and when they should not be used. A recommended textbook to help you with this is provided in the annotated reading list.

Oxygen therapy and nebulisers

You will come across various oxygen delivery systems and devices on both medical and surgical wards. You need to be aware of how to administer oxygen as you will be expected to alter the delivery rate based on patients' vital sign results, mentioned before. Remember that both oxygen and nebulisers are medications and need to be prescribed (Dougherty and West-Oram, 2015).

Patient admission

A patient can be admitted to the ward from another department within the hospital or they can be transferred from another hospital. They can also be admitted for a procedure and that would mean they are admitted directly to the ward from home (this occurs most commonly on surgical wards). There is a certain amount of documentation to go through and complete when a patient is admitted. Completing a patient's admission documentation provides a good opportunity for you to learn and practise various assessments in line with ward policy. You are also likely to see a nurse formulating care plans at this stage. These include written care plans in nursing notes or generated by a computer system, both of which provide valuable learning opportunities for you.

Assessment

You will observe and participate in numerous assessments when it comes to patient care, such as skin assessment, pressure ulcer assessment or nutritional assessment, as well as risk assessment associated with devices used in the delivery of care. You may also come across personal risk assessments when working in highly specialised areas or with harmful substances.

Patient discharge

You will be involved under supervision in the coordination of the processes involved in managing the safe discharge of a patient. Patients can be discharged home, to another hospital or another care setting (like nursing or residential home, respite care or a hospice). There are numerous learning opportunities here, such as completion of the required documentation, liaising with other members of the team both inside and outside the hospital (for instance, district nurses, GP practice, care home staff, social services). You will be directly involved under supervision in the organisation of medications ready for discharge as well as organising transport for the patient if required.

Moving and handling

You will come across a variety of moving and handling procedures across all ward settings. These include assistance in repositioning a patient who is immobile, helping a patient out into a chair or assisting while walking and the use of specialist equipment.

You need to make sure that you always follow the up-to-date training you will have received from your employer in order to provide safe patient care as well as look after your own health when it comes to moving and handling. Never volunteer to use equipment if you are not familiar with the way it operates, even if it is something as simple as an electric patient bed.

Hydration and nutrition

There are a number of tasks you will be involved in order to meet a patient's nutritional needs. These include encouraging a patient to eat and drink, assisting with feeding, documentation of food and fluid intake as well as administration of artificial feeding when patients cannot take food by mouth (e.g. through nasogastric (NG) route).

Patient comfort measures

Patient comfort measures include assisting patients with personal hygiene needs, grooming, helping with getting dressed, assisting a patient to the toilet or with the use of a urinal, bedpan or commode. It is important to remember the simple things – helping patients with mouth care and allowing patients time to wash their hands after using their toilet – all of which provide valuable learning for you.

Collection of samples

It will be your responsibility to collect various biological samples from patients. Examples include sputum, blood, faeces, urine and swabs (for instance, of a suspected infected wound).

Deteriorating patient

As you will be involved in monitoring of patients' vital signs, assisting them in their personal hygiene and mobility, as well as meeting their nutritional and hydration needs, you are in a unique position to identify very quickly if a patient deteriorates or is at risk of deteriorating. Your responsibility will be to act appropriately by raising the alarm to alert other staff for help, and attend to the patient (NMC, 2018d). You will get involved in the subsequent events in patient care such as performing cardiopulmonary resuscitation (CPR). You should make it your priority when arriving at each new hospital ward placement to identify the location of resuscitation equipment (also called resuscitation trolley) and become familiar with the resuscitation policy and procedures, as they may differ slightly between each area.

Documentation

You will have numerous opportunities to practise documentation of care delivered to patients based on all of the learning opportunities mentioned above. This can be done in a patient's notes, or on the computer in areas where documentation has been digitalised.

Activity 7.3   Reflection

Now that you have a brief overview of the learning opportunities available on the hospital ward, revisit your PAD and try to identify the proficiencies that could be achieved and assessed in that setting. You may wish to discuss this with your PA or PA during your initial interview when you start your placement.

An outline answer is given at the end of the chapter.

Having discussed learning opportunities on hospital wards, we will now focus on specific learning applicable to medical and surgical wards.

Learning on medical wards

Most patients on general medicine wards are admitted through A&E departments with a range of medical conditions, such as an exacerbation of a long-term condition (e.g. diabetes), a newly diagnosed acute illness or an infection. Medical wards provide services to adults of all ages across a wide range of specialties and the majority of patients will have complex care needs.

You will be given the chance to develop your skills in all of the patient care tasks discussed above. The following are some learning opportunities specific to the general medical wards.

Infection control measures

It is everybody's responsibility to try to prevent the spread of infection in the hospital. Acquiring an infection can put the life of vulnerable patients in our care at risk

(NMC, 2018d). When in hospital, even if patients are not admitted due to infection, they are at risk of developing one, and this is called a healthcare-associated infection (HCAI) (Dougherty and West-Oram, 2015). These could include, but are not limited to, respiratory infections, sepsis, gastrointestinal infections (e.g. *Clostridium difficile* (*C. diff*) or norovirus), wound or blood stream infections. In order to provide safe care you will need to adhere to infection control measures and guidelines (like hand hygiene) and wear appropriate personal protective equipment (PPE) as instructed. You will care for patients who have developed infections in single isolation rooms, while other areas practise 'cohort isolation' at the bedside. This means looking after a group of patients with the same infection grouped together in an open bay (particularly during an outbreak, when resources do not allow for individual isolation). You can also get involved in the decontamination processes of the area once a patient has been discharged.

Skin care

Due to an ageing population, a considerable proportion of patients on medical wards are elderly (Smith et al., 2014). Age puts patients at risk of developing pressure ulcers due to multiple co-morbidities, loss of collagen, decreased mobility, increased risk of incontinence and issues with nutrition and/or hydration (Jaul et al., 2018). Appropriate and frequent skin assessment is crucial in the prevention of development of pressure ulcers. If pressure ulcers do develop, you will be involved in their assessment and management, which could involve choosing appropriate dressings. You will be encouraged to consider not only the treatment of the wound, but also the causes of the pressure ulcer, like nutrition, hydration and appropriate skin care, including cleansing and moisturising (Kottner et al., 2019).

Continence

Issues with continence can have a direct impact on a patient's skin. Incontinence puts patients at greater risk of developing pressure ulcers. This is caused by a combination of factors, such as prolonged periods of moisture applied to the skin and damaging effects of waste products present in the urine (Peate, 2019). It is important not to presume that every elderly patient is incontinent, therefore effective communication and assessment are crucial. Once you have established that a patient needs assistance in this area, you will be involved in choosing the appropriate continence products and supporting the patient in their toileting needs.

Co-morbidity (also called multimorbidity)

Due to advancements in healthcare, medications and technology, we are now living longer. This means that we are also living with multiple conditions that we are usually able to manage on our own (Payne, 2016). When patients with multiple co-morbidities are admitted to a medical ward, you will be required to meet their complex care needs. This is the perfect opportunity to learn about the assessment and management of long-term conditions, and you will be able to link the theory you learnt at university regarding anatomy and physiology as well as pathophysiology of various diseases. This will also be the perfect opportunity for you to demonstrate your knowledge of holistic patient care (NMC, 2018a). Some conditions that patients are admitted with include, but are not limited to, Crohn's disease, diabetes, irritable bowel syndrome (IBS), colitis, arthritis, hypertension, epilepsy, respiratory infections (chest infection, pneumonia) or chronic pain. Patients suffering from a stroke, cancer or cardiac conditions will be admitted to specialist areas in the hospital; however if this is not the primary reason for their admission, they could also present to the general medical ward.

Polypharmacy

When patients suffer from multiple conditions (as addressed in the previous paragraph), they are likely to require the use of multiple medicines in order to help manage those conditions. This is called polypharmacy (Payne, 2016). Caring for patients on multiple medications provides a valuable learning opportunity for you to consider how drugs might interact with each other, or how certain drugs work together.

Student tip 7.3

Whenever I was placed on a medical ward, I would choose one patient I was looking after who required multiple medications to manage their various conditions. I would take note of all of the medications and explore them in relation to the patient's care plan. I paid particular attention to how the medications interact with each other. I would also check if all medications were taken at the same time, which ones were taken on an empty stomach and which were required to be taken with the main meal.

Angelito, Year 1 NA student

Complex discharge planning

As mentioned previously, you will have the opportunity to get involved in a discharge-planning process. In the case of a patient with complex care needs the discharge process is more complicated, takes more time and will include a wider multidisciplinary team (MDT) and, most importantly, the patient's family and caregivers (Rowe et al., 2020). Therefore this provides an opportunity for you to engage with the MDT and work to ensure the safe discharge of a patient with complex care needs.

End-of-life care

The majority of people in the UK die in hospital, therefore you are likely to come across patients requiring end-of-life care on a medical ward (Rowe et al., 2020). Providing end-of-life care is a difficult experience for any healthcare professional, so you need to make sure you are supported before you can care for the patient and their relatives. You will be involved in providing comfort measures, communication with patient and family, transfer to home or hospice as well as preparation of the deceased patient for transfer to mortuary. For further guidance on this, see Chapter 9.

Having discussed learning opportunities on medical wards, we will now look at the members of the MDT specific to those areas.

The multidisciplinary team specific to the medical ward

You will have the opportunity to work with specialist teams such as:

- palliative care nurse
- tissue viability nurse (TVN)
- alcohol liaison nurse
- stroke clinical nurse specialist
- pain clinical nurse specialist
- continence clinical nurse specialist
- speech and language therapist (SaLT)
- occupational therapist (OT)
- physiotherapist
- infection control nurse specialist
- outreach team
- complex discharge team

Activity 7.4   Critical thinking

When in placement, revisit the above list of members of the MDT, as well as the learning opportunities discussed above. Can you identify which aspects of patient care each member will be involved in?

As this activity is based on your own critical thinking, there is no outline answer at the end of the chapter.

Dementia care of patients in a hospital setting

Around 850,000 people are living with dementia in the UK at the moment (Dementia UK, 2021) and you will certainly come across a patient in your care suffering from this condition, regardless of the type they were diagnosed with. You may encounter those experiences when on general medical wards because patients are admitted for other reasons, or they can be inpatients because of the early onset of dementia (when they have not been officially diagnosed yet). It can often be difficult to provide optimal care for patients with dementia on a busy medical ward. Therefore, a number of hospitals have now created specialist dementia wards, with an adapted environment to suit the needs of patients (Alzheimer's Society, 2021).

It is important to strive to provide the best care possible when looking after a patient with dementia on the general medical ward, even if specialist adjustments are not available. You may already be familiar with schemes that are being rolled out across

UK hospitals to support patients, staff and family members/carers. An example is the *This is Me* tool, a simple leaflet containing the details of patients who are unable to communicate their needs. Another is the *Butterfly Scheme*, which acts as an active symbol showing that support is needed, and extends further to any patient suffering from confusion, regardless of dementia diagnosis.

Having looked at the medical wards, we can now move on to exploring learning available to students on surgical wards.

Learning on surgical wards

Patients can be admitted to a surgical ward for an elective (planned) or emergency surgery. The outcomes and recovery time will differ depending on the type of admission or surgery, and these will be specific, alongside familiar learning opportunities that can be achieved on highly specialised units like orthopaedic or transplant wards.

Case study: Darek

You are currently on placement on one of the surgical wards and Darek is a patient due to undergo a Hartmann's procedure in the afternoon. You have been allocated to work alongside your PS to prepare the patient for surgery. Darek is otherwise fit and healthy. He is currently nil by mouth (NBM) and therefore an infusion of intravenous (IV) fluids is in progress. Darek is quite anxious about the surgery as he has had other procedures before and does not deal with pain very well.

Activity 7.5   Critical thinking

Make a list of the preoperative checks, assessments and procedures that will be undertaken for this patient before he can be transferred to the operating theatre.

An outline answer is given at the end of the chapter.

Pre- and post-operative surgical/nursing care

This will involve a number of assessments and safety checks before the patient is deemed safe to undergo surgery. Before a patient is taken to the operating theatre, you will be involved in tasks like carrying out an electrocardiogram (ECG), vital signs, preoperative checklist, application of anti-embolism stockings and administration of preoperative medication. Before the patient comes back from theatre, you will prepare the bed space, organise equipment required (e.g. infusion drip stands and volumetric pumps) and make sure safety equipment is in working order (e.g. wall-mounted suction and oxygen). Once the patient returns from surgery, you will be participating in monitoring of vital signs at regular intervals with particular attention to consciousness level, monitoring and documentation of fluid input and output, monitoring of any drains and wounds and comfort measures like mouth care and repositioning.

Postoperative vital signs monitoring

Regular monitoring and accurate record of patient observation following ward policy are crucial in order to maintain the patient's safety. Apart from vital signs, you could be performing a quick ABCDE assessment, further discussed in Chapter 8.

Complex and simple wound care

Surgical wards give you the perfect opportunity to develop knowledge in the area of wound management. You will be able to assess and manage some very common wounds following a surgical incision to the hip, knee, neck or abdomen, for example. These could be closed using sutures or clips and covered with a simple dressing. Wounds that are more complex will usually require input of a TVN and may necessitate a more complicated dressing, a number of dressings or more advanced wound management systems. You may also be involved in stoma care (following bowel surgery). Whether simple or complex, all wounds put patients at risk of developing an infection, therefore an aseptic (clean) technique needs to be implemented at all times when changing the dressing.

Pain assessment and management

Patients are likely to suffer from pain before surgery as they are awaiting a remedy to their problem, after surgery following manipulation of tissues and due to the wound as a result of the procedure. You will be involved in administration of simple analgesia, while nurses will assist patients with IV medications and opioids. You will become familiar with the common pain assessment tools as well as other non-pharmaceutical pain-relieving measures.

Activity 7.6   Critical thinking

Considering the above information, and looking back at the case study of Darek, think about pain management following his surgery. What could be some of the challenges in pain assessment and management of Darek? Is there anything that could be done before he undergoes the procedure?

An outline answer is given at the end of the chapter.

Fluid and nutritional management

Following surgery, patients are usually encouraged to introduce a light diet gradually. Contraindications to oral intake will be documented in the post-op surgical notes, and communicated during the handover. When encouraging patients to drink and then eat, you need to be mindful of the effects of surgery and analgesia on the body. Patients may be nauseous or vomiting. It is crucial to anticipate this and prepare appropriate equipment to be able to assist the patient. You also need to pay particular attention to the patient's urine output, particularly if an indwelling urinary catheter is in place, as any decrease in urine could indicate that the patient is deteriorating.

Assistance with mobility

Following most types of surgery, early mobility is encouraged in order to avoid complications such as a chest infection, pressure ulcer and constipation. After more complex surgery, the patient will have to be assessed by a physiotherapist before being transferred following bedrest; however, on most occasions you should be able to assist them on your own or with another member of staff. You need to bear in mind some of the factors mentioned before, like nausea and vomiting, as well as the patient's pain.

Enhanced recovery pathway

Surgical wards will implement these pathways for patients undergoing minor elective procedures. These are patient-centred pathways based on the latest available evidence, relying on the involvement of the MDT and devised for each speciality. The aim is to facilitate recovery and hopefully shorten hospital stay by empowering patients to be involved in the recovery process and optimise their physiological function (Paton et al., 2014).

Transfer of patients to an intensive care unit (ICU)

As mentioned before, your role will be to assess the patient according to the treatment they are receiving and to be able to recognise and escalate when their condition deteriorates. If that happens and the patient would benefit from closer monitoring on the ICU, you will be involved in preparation of the patient, the transfer, as well as communication with the patient's family.

Now that we have discussed some of the most common learning opportunities on the surgical ward, we can look at the members of the MDT with whom you may be working closely.

Activity 7.7   Critical thinking

Think back to our case study and the patient, Darek. Which members of the MDT will be involved in his care? What learning could you be gaining from working with those team members?

An outline answer is given at the end of the chapter.

The multidisciplinary team specific to the surgical ward

You will have the opportunity to work with specialist teams such as:

- pain clinical nurse specialist
- stoma care nurse specialist
- dietician
- physiotherapist
- TVN
- surgeon and the surgical team of doctors
- anaesthetist
- outreach team

During your placement, talk with your PA or PS to arrange some time to shadow the above MDT members as this will be a valuable learning experience for you.

Chapter summary

This chapter began with an overview of everyday practice on the adult hospital ward, including daily ward routine, members of the MDT and the usual tasks that students will be involved in, which will allow them to meet most of their proficiencies in the PAD. Learning opportunities on the medical ward were explored, with additional focus on dementia settings. The chapter concluded with a discussion on learning available on surgical wards, and discussion of the most commonly performed tasks irrespective of surgical speciality.

Activities: brief outline answers

Activity 7.1 Evidence-based practice and research

Answers will vary depending on the local Trust and whether the hospital is general or a single speciality. Sometimes it is very easy to guess the speciality as it will be given away in the name (e.g. 'Surgical ward 1'), but at times it may not be that obvious. Try to access the Trust's webpage and search for a ward directory. This could help as it usually includes a brief description of services provided by each area.

Activity 7.2 Critical thinking

You will be discussing those proficiencies at university during one of the Year 1 modules. You will be familiar with important Nursing and Midwifery Council

(NMC) guidance on nursing documentation and you are likely to discuss the Caldicott Principles (Department of Health, 2013) that safeguard patients' right to confidentiality. You may find the House of Commons Library document, available in the annotated useful websites on the next page very useful as it summarises the relevant Acts of Parliament (e.g. Data Protection Act 1998, Access to Health Records Act 1990 and many other relevant legislation).

Activity 7.3 Reflection

Most proficiencies in the PAD in both years of your programme are easily achievable on general adult hospital wards. Try to familiarise yourself with proficiencies before each ward placement starts, and group them in meaningful clusters to make the best of your learning.

Activity 7.5 Critical thinking

Preoperative preparation will include a variety of nursing activities. You may have thought about the patient's appearance to start with, and the fact that he needs to change into a hospital gown. Safety checks need to be performed, and all documentation needs to be in place and accurate. This will involve communication with the patient, family/carers and other professionals. Use the paragraphs following the activity, as well as the resource on surgical nursing procedures (example available in annotated further reading list), to model your answer.

Activity 7.6 Critical thinking

It is important that during patient assessment a patient's anxieties around pain are established and managed before he undergoes the procedure. This can be done by explaining pain management options with Darek, asking him what strategies usually work for him (both pharmacological and non-pharmacological) and he could also be referred to the Pain Management Team for further advice.

Activity 7.7 Critical thinking

Firstly you need to explore what a Hartmann's procedure is. It is a bowel surgery (resection of the colon) and the patient is very likely to require formation of an end colostomy (also called a stoma). This means that one of the first clinical nurse specialists Darek will see before surgery is a stoma nurse, who will assess him for the position of the stoma and prepare him physically and mentally for what care of stoma and stoma bag entails. You will be able to observe excellent communication skills during this assessment, and the nurse is likely to allow plenty of time for the patient to process the information.

Darek will be seen by the anaesthetist before surgery, and this will be the perfect opportunity for you to explore the principles of informed written consent. This could be taking place in collaboration with the patient's surgeon. This case study will also require an input from a dietician, as type of bowel movement will vary in the early stages following surgery and the patient will have to be advised on how to manage this with appropriate diet. Depending on the outcome and complexity of the surgery, the patient could require input from all the other members of the team mentioned in this chapter. From Activity 7.6 you are also now aware of the importance of the pain management team. Make sure you volunteer in any activities that require MDT involvement as these are invaluable learning opportunities.

Annotated useful websites

Free resources on the Royal College of Nursing (RCN) website related to end-of-life care, focusing on effective communication and holistic patient care as well as ethical issues: https://rcni.com/hosted-content/rcn/fundamentals-of-end-of-life-care/getting-started

A useful summary of the legislation and guidance relating to medical records prepared by the House of Commons Library: www.nhsconfed.org/resources/2015/10/legislation-and-guidance-relating-to-medical-records-explained-by-house-of-commons-library

Annotated further reading

Roulston, C. and Davies, M. (2021) *Medicines Management for Nursing Associates.* London: SAGE.

This book will help you develop your skills in effective management and administration of medicines.

Smith, A., Kisiel, M. and Radford, M. (2016) *Oxford Handbook of Surgical Nursing.* New York: Oxford University Press.

An essential resource useful to healthcare professionals who look after patients before and after surgery.

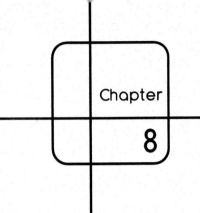

Acute care settings

Cariona Flaherty and Sinead Mehigan

NMC STANDARDS OF PROFICIENCY FOR REGISTERED NURSING ASSOCIATES (NMC, 2018A)

This chapter will address the following platforms and proficiencies:

Platform 3: Provide and monitor care

At the point of registration, the nursing associate will be able to:

3.7   demonstrate and apply an understanding of how and when to escalate to the appropriate professional for expert help and advice.

3.8   demonstrate and apply an understanding of how people's needs for safety, dignity, privacy, comfort and sleep can be met.

3.11 demonstrate the ability to recognise when a person's condition has improved or deteriorated by undertaking health monitoring. Interpret, promptly respond, share findings and escalate as needed.

Platform 4: Working in teams

At the point of registration, the nursing associate will be able to:

4.1   demonstrate an awareness of the roles, responsibilities and scope of practice of different members of the nursing and interdisciplinary team, and their own role within it.

4.3   understand and apply the principles of human factors and environmental factors when working in teams.

Platform 6: Contributing to integrated care

At the point of registration, the nursing associate will be able to:

6.1   understand the roles of the different providers of health and care. Demonstrate the ability to work collaboratively and in partnership with professionals from different agencies in interdisciplinary teams.

Chapter aims

By the end of this chapter you should be able to:

- identify ways to prepare for a placement in an acute care setting.
- discuss learning when undertaking a placement in Accident and Emergency (A&E) or Intensive Care Unit (ICU / critical care).
- identify transferable and specialist skills that can be learnt when undertaking an A&E or ICU placement.
- describe learning from undertaking a placement in theatres, with a focus on perioperative care, the anaesthetic room and recovery.

Introduction

Price (2019, p. 43) highlighted that 'clinical placements are important for students, because they provide an authentic experience of day-to-day clinical practice, and because students can learn from nurses' clinical reasoning' while on placement. However, clinical placements can often be quite a daunting experience for students due to the unpredictable nature of clinical environments, especially within acute care settings. ICU, A&E and theatres provide specialist clinical experience for students, and often students can encounter opportunistic learning as a result of the rapidly changing acuity of patients within these settings. Placements within acute care settings can happen throughout your programme, and for some, acute care settings may be their normal place of work. Theory related to caring for acutely unwell and complex patients will occur across Years 1 and 2; however the complexity of this learning will increase as you progress from Year 1 to Year 2. This chapter will discuss the learning you can gain from undertaking placements in acute care settings with a focus on ICU, A&E and theatres. This discussion will include identifying ways in which you can prepare for acute care placements as well as acknowledging key specialist and transferable skills.

Activity 8.1 Reflection

Normally in Year 1 you would learn about clinical skills such as monitoring of patient vital signs; blood pressure, pulse, temperature, respiratory rate and saturations. As you move into Year 2 the modules you undertake increase in complexity. For example, in Year 1 you learn about anatomy and physiology, and often pathophysiology. In Year 2 you learn how to apply such learning to increasingly complex clinical scenarios. Take a look at the modules you will complete in Years 1 and 2 of your programme. Make a list of what modules and content you will be able to draw learning from to use when you are undertaking placements within acute care settings.

As this activity is based on your own reflection, no outline answer is provided at the end of the chapter.

Preparing for placements in acute care settings

Having looked at each of your modules and identified learning which you can use to support you while undertaking a placement in an acute care setting, it is now important to identify how you can prepare before such placements begin. Day-Calder (2017) suggests these are the following steps you should take before placement begins:

- *Research the clinical area*: This can be done with a Google search of the hospital and clinical area. ICU, A&E and theatres are specialist clinical areas and very different in terms of layout, equipment and staffing. Therefore it is essential that you do some research into these areas prior to starting placement.
- *Arrange a pre-placement visit*: ICU, A&E and theatres are very different in terms of setting and environment when compared to ward or community settings. Therefore it is advisable and important that you book in a pre-placement visit. This can help to relieve some of the anxieties you may have.
- *Think back on previous learning and how this can support you*: Activity 8.1 asked you to review learning from your programme that you can use to support you when undertaking placements in acute care settings. It is also worthwhile reflecting back on previous placements – what went well, what did not go well – and then use this to plan for your upcoming placements. For example, you might not have organised a pre-placement visit and when starting a placement you ended up getting lost and went to the wrong department. Therefore, for this placement use this experience to ensure you do book in a pre-placement visit.
- *Think about learning objectives*: When undertaking placements in acute care settings you need to think carefully about specific learning objectives. Most students entering such placement areas will want to learn about invasive mechanical ventilation (MV), but this would be classed as an unrealistic expectation. Learning about MV takes a number of years and requires specialist training. In addition, MV would be seen as a specialist skill as opposed to a transferable skill. However, learning about non-invasive ventilation such as continuous positive airway pressure (CPAP) could be seen as a transferable skill because CPAP is now being used more frequently outside ICU environments. Shirey (2009, p. 128) defined transferable skills as 'skills, abilities and personal attributes that an individual can use in a wide range of activities. Transferable skills represent a potpourri of skills that an individual may have learnt in academic life but fine-tuned through work experience, daily living and broad personal engagement'. When undertaking a clinical placement you need to consider learning objectives in the context of transferable skills; for example, MV will only ever be used in ICU, A&E or theatre – making this a specialist skill. In comparison, assessment of an acutely ill patient is a skill that can be used in any clinical setting – therefore making this skill transferable. For more information on developing learning objectives for your placement refer to Chapter 2.

- *Think about your upcoming assessments*: As mentioned previously, teaching in relation to caring for the acutely unwell and complex patients will usually take place in Year 2 of your programme, which may coincide with placements in ICU, A&E and theatre. You need to consider what assessments you have coming up and how undertaking placements in acute care settings can provide support for these assessments. For example, you will have to undertake a drug calculation exam during your programme. ICU, A&E and theatres deal with complex drug administration and calculations, thus providing an excellent opportunity for you to practise your drug calculations.

The above steps are some things you can consider in order to prepare for placement in acute care settings. Chapter 1 provides extensive examples of how you can prepare for and get the most out of clinical placements. If you haven't done so already, look at Chapter 1 now.

Learning from ICU (critical care)

Having considered preparation for placement, this section will introduce learning from ICU. Critical care units are where very sick patients are taken care of and receive specialist, highly technical treatment. On the first day of your placement you will have a comprehensive induction. This will include introducing you to the multidisciplinary team (MDT), showing you around the ICU, explaining staffing levels and patient levels, as well as emergency procedures.

Nurse-to-patient ratio in ICU

Staffing in ICU differs from any other area and is dependent on the acuity of patients. The acuity of a patient is identified through various levels:

- *Level 0* – Patients whose needs can be met through normal care in an acute hospital, and are normally cared for at ward level.
- *Level 1* – Patients at risk of their condition deteriorating, or those recently relocated from higher levels of care whose needs can be met on an acute ward with advice and support.
- *Level 2* – Patients requiring more detailed observation or interventions, including single-organ support, postoperative care or those stepping down from Level 3. Patients in Level 2 are often referred to as 'high dependency' and the nurse-to-patient ratio is normally one nurse to two patients.
- *Level 3* – Patients requiring advanced respiratory support (MV) or support for at least two organs, or complex multiorgan failure. The nurse-to-patient ratio is normally one nurse to one patient.

(Dutton and Finch, 2018, p. 3)

It is worth noting that the nurse-to-patient ratio is not static, and may change in order to deal with the increasing number of patients requiring critical care, among other things. Therefore if you undertake placements in critical care be aware that the nurse-to-patient ratio may be subject to change.

The multidisciplinary team in ICU

ICU units operate and function through teamwork with a variety of healthcare professionals from the MDT. When you are on placement in ICU you will have the opportunity to work with various professionals and this will add to a wider learning experience. This could in fact become one of your learning outcomes. Alongside working with other professionals, you will be welcomed to attend ward rounds and MDT meetings where the care of complex and long-term patients is comprehensively discussed. The MDT include:

- doctor (consultant, registrar, senior house office, house officer, medical student)
- nurse (matron, senior sister, junior sister, band 5, Nursing Associate (NA), student nurse, student NA)
- physiotherapist
- occupational therapist
- speak and language therapist
- dietitian
- microbiologist
- infection control nurse

During your placement, talk with your practice assessor (PA) / practice supervisor (PS) to arrange a time when you can shadow some of the above MDT members; this will be a valuable learning experience for you.

Learning opportunities in ICU

As previously mentioned, when considering learning you need to think about transferable skills. Such skills include:

- *Communication*: You will encounter patients who cannot speak due to having a tracheostomy or being intubated. This can be used as a learning opportunity to consider how you may adapt your communication skills to meet the needs of patients who cannot speak. In addition, you will get to experience how nurses speak to relatives, either to deliver an update on the progress of the patient or to comfort families when patients are receiving end-of-life care.
- *Handover*: ICU handovers are complex because of the acuity of patients. Nurses tend to use the Resuscitation Council UK ABCDE framework (2015) in the handover of patients. Although in principle this is an assessment framework, it can also be used to provide a comprehensive handover ensuring all bodily systems are covered.
- *Monitoring of vital signs*: You will have already gained experience of undertaking observations from previous placements and you can use this as a transferable skill during your placement in ICU. Do remember that in ICU observations are normally hourly and are very closely monitored and managed.
- *Patient assessment*: As previously mentioned, the ABCDE assessment framework (Resuscitation Council UK, 2015) is utilised to assess and in the handover of patients in ICU. This framework should not be new to you, and learning on this normally begins in Year 1 of your study. A placement in ICU provides an

excellent opportunity for you to practise and refine your ability to assess a patient comprehensively using the ABCDE assessment framework.

Other learning includes:

- *Care of devices*: drains, catheters, intravenous (IV) lines and nasogastric (NG) tubes. Although you will not be involved in administering IVs, you can learn how to monitor an IV line for infection.
- *Insertion of devices*: You will have the opportunity to observe insertion of a variety of devices, such as a tracheostomy, central line, arterial line, haemofiltration line and NG tube.
- *Documentation*: ICUs are in the main moving their patient documentation online, therefore all observations and documentation will be completed online using a variety of systems. This provides the opportunity for you to enhance your digital literacy skills – a key tenet of the NMC (2018a).
- *Postoperative care*: ICUs are normally located close to theatres, and patients are often transferred from recovery for further one-to-one care in ICU. You will learn how to care for and monitor a patient postoperatively.
- *Complex patient positioning*: In ICU patients with severe respiratory illness are often placed in different positions which you will not have seen before. Some patients will be placed on a turning mattress, which will change the patient's position from right to left at various intervals. In addition patients may be placed in a prone position to improve oxygenation. Prone positioning is face down, and requires a highly skilled team to manage MV and turn the patient safely.
- *Transfer of a patient*: ICU patients are often transferred to other areas within hospitals for magnetic resonance imaging (MRI), X-ray, interventional radiology or surgery. Transferring a critically unwell patient is complex, requires several MDT professionals as well as numerous drugs and pieces of equipment, and provides a useful learning opportunity for students during placement.

The above points are not exhaustive and you will of course have any number of opportunities to immerse yourself in learning routine nursing care, such as wound care, mouth care, hygiene needs and pressure area care, among others. I would

Activity 8.2   Evidence-based practice

The section on learning opportunities in ICU mentioned the ABCDE assessment framework. Using the following link, review the ABCDE assessment and take time to learn the various components. This will ensure you can use the ABCDE assessment during an ICU placement and provide an opportunity for you to refine this transferable skill.

The ABCDE approach: www.resus.org.uk/library/2015-resuscitation-guidelines/abcde-approach

An outline answer is given at the end of the chapter.

encourage you to think widely and use your placement in ICU to consider how caring for complex and acutely unwell patients fits into your learning and how you can utilise the experience throughout your career. Additionally, while undertaking placement in ICU you will have the opportunity to learn about various illnesses and often you will encounter cardiac arrest situations. Activity 8.2 asks you to engage with evidence-based practice with a view to supporting you for placements in ICU.

Learning from A&E (Emergency Department)

Activity 8.2 can be used in all acute care settings, especially in A&E where acutely unwell patients are regularly admitted. This section will look at learning that can take place by exploring each area in A&E separately. A&E areas provide a multitude of learning opportunities for students on clinical placements. This is mainly because of the unpredictability of patients on admission and due to the various areas within A&E. The three main areas in A&E are resuscitation, majors and minors. Let's look at each area individually:

Resuscitation

In the resuscitation room you will learn how various members of the MDT work together to manage complex, acute and often life-threatening or life-limiting situations. As a student you will often take on the role of observer, finding a position where you are not in the way and watching how patients are managed. Your PS/PA may ask you to get some equipment that is needed, but in the main your role will be to observe. Observing situations within the resuscitation room provides a unique opportunity for reflection and learning by observation.

Majors

Bowen (2017) identifies 'majors' as an area where patients require assessment, investigation and often diagnosis which will likely result in hospital admission. The learning from this area includes assessment, history taking, clinical investigations such as urinalysis, bloods, X-ray or computed tomography (CT) scan. All of this is similar to learning (which again is transferable) that can take place in ICU and theatre.

Minors

Minors is for patients who need treatment but do not require hospital admission. Admissions to this area are normally for minor sprains, breaks, cuts or minor infections such as urinary tract infection. Assessment and treatment are normally carried out by advanced nurse practitioners or emergency doctors. You can learn how to assess and treat minor conditions in this area such as applying bandages or slings for sprains.

The multidisciplinary team in A&E

As well as the above three areas you will have the opportunity to work with specialist teams such as:

- alcohol liaison team
- social worker
- paramedic
- safeguarding / domestic violence team
- clinical nurse specialist
- plaster nurse / doctor
- research nurse
- radiographer
- mental health liaison team
- physiotherapist
- occupational therapist
- hospital discharge team

Activity 8.3   Critical thinking

Looking at the above list of specialist teams within A&E, identify what each professional does, and what learning you could take from spending time during a placement with each. Remember to consider transferable skills.

As this activity is based on your own critical thinking activity in preparation for undertaking a placement in A&E, no outline answer is given at the end of the chapter.

Transferable and specialist learning from A&E

Activity 8.3 asks you to identify transferable skills that you could develop when working with various specialist teams in A&E. To help you think about this, the following list provides examples of transferable and specialist learning that can take place when undertaking a placement in A&E.

Transferable A&E skills

- patient assessment and the nursing process
- documentation and reporting of patient care
- communication – verbal and non-verbal
- team work
- time management
- infection control procedures
- safe discharge home or to a ward setting
- patient discharge
- pain management
- pressure area care
- wound care and dressings

Specialist A&E skills

- principles of application of plaster of Paris
- CPR
- minor injuries – assessment and management
- overdose and poisoning
- trauma care
- mental health issues – dealing with them and seeking support
- airway management
- primary and secondary surveys

This list is not exhaustive but does provide scope for thinking about what you will learn when undertaking a placement in A&E. Now let us consider learning from theatres.

Learning from theatres

Perioperative placement

This section focuses on the learning opportunities you may expect when contributing to patient care within a perioperative setting. The operating department can sometimes feel like an overwhelming and frightening place, which bears little relation to anywhere you have worked before. It also seems to be populated with a vast number of staff who are involved in caring for the patient. Even if you decide that you never want to work there, hopefully you will gain useful insights into the patient's experience of surgery. These insights should give you knowledge to enable you to deliver more informed care to your patients as an NA in the future. You will find that your knowledge of patient safety issues and MDT working in particular will be enhanced through working here. A placement in this area will also allow you to:

- gain an insight into surgery
- improve your pre- and postoperative patient care
- gain a better insight into anatomy and physiology
- improve your skills in aseptic technique
- improve your skills at managing a patient's airway
- appreciate the value of multiprofessional teamwork

Case study: Gloria

You are an NA student on a practice learning opportunity in the operating department and are observing practice in the anaesthetic room. A patient, Gloria, has just been brought to the anaesthetic room; according to the theatre list, she is having her right hip replaced. The operating theatre is very busy, due to several emergency cases added before Gloria's case. You are waiting with Gloria for the anaesthetist to arrive. Gloria says that she is glad she is having this surgery, as she has had pain in her left hip for such a long time. You are concerned because it seems that there may have been some miscommunication between members of the healthcare team.

Gloria's incident above is an excellent example of the importance of clear communication, and raises issues of patient safety that you may encounter in the perioperative setting. We will refer back to this case study, and address concerns identified further later in the chapter.

The remainder of this section will be divided into three parts, reflecting the patient's journey through the perioperative setting – preoperatively, in the anaesthetic room; intraoperatively, in the operating theatre; and postoperatively, in the recovery room. As part of your placement, you are likely to be given opportunities to rotate through all three areas.

Anaesthetic room

On the day of surgery, the anaesthetist and member of the surgical team will visit the patient to carry out final checks and ensure that the patient is ready for surgery. A patient like Gloria will have been prepared for surgery by the ward staff and will come to the anaesthetic room with her notes and consent form. In Gloria's case, you noticed that there was a difference between what she thought she was having (surgery on her left hip), and what was on the theatre list (surgery on the right hip). One of the measures that perioperative teams have put in place to ensure a 'never event', such as performing an operation on the wrong hip, is to adopt 'Five Steps to Safer Surgery', developed and promoted by the World Health Organization (2008). Following this system, surgical teams use a series of steps and checks at each stage of the patient's perioperative journey, to minimise any risk to their safety. One of these steps involves a surgical team, including anaesthetists, surgeons, nursing and other support staff, meeting for a pre-session 'huddle', or team briefing. At this stage, each patient on the list is discussed, and any specific queries about patients or final planning is agreed on. The next stage is to check the patient into the anaesthetic room. If you are worried about an anomaly between what is written on the theatre list and what the patient tells you, you should raise your concerns with the nursing and anaesthetic staff.

Depending on the type of surgery that patients undergo, they may have different types of anaesthetic. If they are having major surgery, they will usually be given a general anaesthetic, where they are 'put to sleep' for the duration of a procedure. Having a general anaesthetic means that a patient may get a combination of drugs – intravenously or administered through their airway, to make them unconscious, to give them pain relief, and, in some instances, to relax their muscles sufficiently to enable surgery to take place. These three parts of a general anaesthetic are sometimes referred to as the 'triad' of anaesthesia.

Other types of anaesthetics that can be used include regional anaesthesia, where a local anaesthetic is administered to a specific region of the body, leading to numbness or pain relief for deeper operations where more extensive numbness is needed. Patients like Gloria can have hip surgery performed using a type of regional anaesthesia called a spinal anaesthetic. Other more minor surgery can be performed using local anaesthesia (where a small area of the body is numbed through injection of an anaesthetic agent like lidocaine, but the patient remains awake) or topical anaesthesia.

Many of the skills that you can develop through being in the anaesthetic area include communication skills, particularly if alleviating a patient's anxiety. Being in this area also gives you excellent opportunities to build on skills you will have developed in your CPR sessions, particularly as they relate to airway management and the use of airway adjuncts.

Operating theatre

Once Gloria has been anaesthetised, she will be transferred to the operating theatre, where she will be prepared for her surgery. The focus of care during this phase is on maintaining her safety, through management of any risks associated with surgery.

Risk of delays due to poor preparation of the area

The scrub and circulating team will carefully prepare the area, ensuring they have all instruments, drapes, swabs and lotions needed. They also spend time ensuring they have the necessary specialised equipment available and set up for use. This might include suction, diathermy, microscopes, air cylinders or lasers, to name a few.

Risk of infection

All members of the surgical team will scrub up for a case using surgical hand-washing techniques and putting on sterile gloves and gowns. All surgical instruments and items used directly during surgery (for example, swabs, sutures, knives) are sterilised before use and kept on a sterile trolley during a procedure. The scrub nurse and surgical team will adopt good aseptic technique to reduce the possibility of introducing infection into the surgical site. Numbers of staff in the operating theatre are limited, and staff are encouraged not to go in and out of the theatre, to reduce disturbance of air.

Risk of items from surgical field being left in the patient

Prior to starting any case in theatres, the scrub nurse will count all instruments, swabs, blades and needles with the circulating staff. This count is recorded, with any additional items, such as swabs, being added to the record as a case progresses. The scrub nurse and circulating staff count all swabs and instruments before any body cavity is closed, to ensure that nothing has been left behind. As part of the WHO Five Steps to Safer Surgery, the surgical team will, as part of their sign-off, ensure that the swab and instrument count is correct.

Risk of injury due to poor positioning

The surgical and anaesthetic team will work together to ensure that a patient is safely positioned for surgery to proceed. For Gloria, this means that she will be positioned on her side, with supports put on her front and back to ensure she does not fall off the table during the procedure.

Risk of developing deep venous thrombosis (DVT)

If a patient has surgery that takes a long time, they are at risk of developing a DVT, due to muscle inactivity during surgery. This means that blood is more likely to collect in the lower limbs. Patients like Gloria are likely to come to theatre wearing compression stockings. Some patients may also have special booties put on prior to surgery. These are attached to a pump, to encourage circulation of blood during a procedure.

Risk of burns due to diathermy

Diathermy is the use of an electrical current to coagulate small blood vessels or cut through tissue. In order to use diathermy safely, it is important that the team apply a diathermy pad to dry, shaved skin that has a good blood supply. This can be on someone's thigh or back. The diathermy pad provides a route for the electricity to return to 'earth' and so minimises the risk of burns to the patient.

During the surgical procedure you will notice the close multidisciplinary teamwork required, with all members of the team using their expertise to ensure that an operation is carried out successfully. This requires clear communication between team members at all times, and a lot of anticipatory actions from the scrub and circulating team, to help respond to any changes that may be needed during a case. You may be given the opportunity to act as the circulator for a case, or scrub alongside a qualified member of staff. If you get this opportunity, it will enhance your understanding and practice in maintaining asepsis, and also provide an excellent view of the surgery and the anatomy involved.

Recovery room

Once surgery is complete, the anaesthetic team will reverse the effects of their anaesthetic agents, so that the patient wakes up. They will then transfer the patient to the recovery room. You will find that this area is more like a ward area. Patients will be kept here, looked after by one nurse, until it is safe to transfer them back to the ward. The emphasis of care in this area continues to be on maintaining patient safety, through close assessment and monitoring.

The first stage of patient care in this area starts before the patient arrives. Each bay will be prepared with all necessary equipment, such as oxygen, a range of oxygen masks, suction, airway adjuncts, monitoring equipment (such as a three-lead electrocardiogram (ECG), blood pressure monitoring and oxygen saturation monitoring). Each recovery area also checks their emergency equipment, resuscitation trolley and drugs on a daily basis.

When a patient is brought into the recovery unit, they must be accompanied by the anaesthetist and a member of the surgical team. The recovery nurse is given a full handover, including patient identity, actual surgery carried out, whether or not there were any complications, if the patient had any pre-existing illnesses that might affect their recovery, anaesthetic drugs and IV fluids administered, if there are any drains inserted, and any specific postoperative instructions.

As the anaesthetic team give their handover, the recovery nurse will make their own systematic assessment of the patient's condition using an adapted ABCDE approach (Hatfield and Tronson, 2009). This involves assessment of:

- *A – airway*: Is the patient able to maintain their own airway? Is their airway clear? The most common problem postoperatively is airway obstruction, due to the patient's tongue falling to the back of their throat. You will know this has happened if you hear the patient snoring. If this happens, the patient should be put on to their side. If this is not possible, you will see staff perform a chin lift. It could also be that a patient has mucus at the back of the throat, leading to a gurgling sound. This can be resolved by gently suctioning secretions from the patient's mouth.

- *B – breathing*: Is the patient breathing normally? Can you see the patient's chest rise and fall gently? Sometimes the drugs used to paralyse a patient's muscles for major surgery may take longer than expected to wear off. The patient may be in a lot of pain, or their respiratory system may still be suppressed from anaesthetic agents or IV analgesics, such as morphine. Normally patients arriving in recovery after a general anaesthetic will be given oxygen, to ensure that their oxygen saturation levels are maintained above 94%.
- *C – circulation and consciousness*: The recovery nurse will take the patient's pulse and blood pressure initially and continue to monitor every 15 minutes. Pain and haemorrhage can both adversely affect a patient's cardiovascular system in the recovery phase. The recovery nurse will also look at a patient's colour – as bluish coloration of a patient's extremities can indicate problems with oxygenation levels. Many patients will have regained consciousness by the time they arrive in the recovery room. However, it is important to be vigilant, particularly after any IV analgesia has been given.
- *D – drugs, drips, dressings and drains*: The anaesthetist should identify what drugs have been given to a patient during surgery. They will also ensure that they have written up prescriptions for analgesics, oxygen, anti-emetics and IV fluids that may be needed by the patient in the postoperative period. This will provide you with opportunities to gain more knowledge and understanding of these drugs. Some patients, if they have lost a lot of blood during surgery, will continue to have an IV infusion in place. The recovery nurse should check on the site and ensure that the IV cannula is secured.

It is important to check a patient's wound dressing when they come out of surgery. You may find that, if there is some blood visible on the dressing, staff mark its extent, so they can gauge the amount of any subsequent bleeding. Although used less often, for some types of surgery, patients will have a drain put in the wound site and attached to a collection device, such as a suction bottle. This is in cases where it is important to drain any blood, pus or other fluid to prevent it accumulating within the body.

- *E – everything else*: This could include: if the patient is a diabetic, do they need an insulin infusion? If they have had orthopaedic surgery, does the surgeon require them to have a splint in place to keep, for example, an operated leg in proper alignment?

The recovery nurse will continue to monitor and record a patient's recovery, taking observations of their respiratory rate, pulse and blood pressure every 15 minutes. The most common problems that patients develop in the recovery room include respiratory problems, pain and nausea and vomiting. Patients will remain in the area until recovery staff are confident that it is safe to transfer them back to the ward area. Patients will be ready for transfer when:

- They are awake, responsive and able to maintain their own airway. Sometimes the recovery nurse will test this by asking a patient to lift and keep their head off the pillow for a short time.
- They are relatively pain-free and have adequate analgesia.
- Their cardiovascular system is stable.

- They have normal respiration and oxygenation levels.
- Their body temperature is within acceptable limits.
- There are no continuing surgical problems (for example, bleeding).
- The recovery staff can give clear instructions to the ward on postoperative care requirements (including oxygen, drugs and fluids).

Ensuring all of the above is in place minimises a patient's risk and ensures that a safe transfer can be achieved.

Chapter summary

This chapter began by providing examples of how to prepare for clinical placements with a particular focus on acute care settings. Learning for ICU was discussed, starting with an overview of the various levels of care, along with identifying the members of the MDT with whom you may be working during a placement in ICU. Learning from A&E focused on three main areas and specialist teams and outlined key transferable and specialist skills which can be learnt while on placement in A&E. The chapter finished with a comprehensive discussion on learning from theatres with a focus on perioperative, intraoperative and postoperative care.

Activities: brief outline answers

Activity 8.2 Reflection

The link provided in this activity takes you to the Resuscitation Council UK website, where you will find a comprehensive approach to undertaking an ABCDE assessment. The ABCDE approach starts by taking you through the underlying principles / first steps, which include personal safety, rapid look, listen, feel, assessing patient responsiveness and monitoring of vital signs. This is all to determine the acuity of the patient and escalation of rapid care if needed. After this the ABCDE assessment approach of *airway, breathing, circulation, disability* and *exposure* is completed in that order. Further information can found on the Resuscitation Council UK website link provided. Learning how to undertake an ABCDE assessment is an essential part of your learning and is seen as a transferable skill regardless of whether you work in an adult, child or mental health setting.

Annotated further reading

Hatfield, A. (2014) *The Complete Recovery Book*, 5th ed. Oxford: Oxford University Press.

This is a very accessible and comprehensive guide to everything you might need to know about helping a patient recover after surgery. You will find that some of the advice can be applied to caring for the surgical patient in the ward area too.

Dutton, H. and Finch, J. (2018) *Acute and Critical Care Nursing at a Glance.* Oxford: Wiley Blackwell.

This book provides an introduction to critical care, and is essential reading when undertaking a placement in ICU.

Armellino, D. (2017) Minimizing Sources of Airborne, Aerosolized, and Contact Contaminants in the OR Environment. *AORN Journal,* 106(6): 494–501.

This gives a detailed account of all possible sources of infection in the operating theatre and advice on how to minimise these.

Gracia, M. (2016) 'Scrubbing up: my first experience as a student nurse in the operating theatre.' *British Journal of Nursing,* 25(11): 621.

If you are offered the opportunity of scrubbing alongside a qualified member of staff, you might find it interesting to compare your experience with this student nurse. Most theatre staff will remember very well their first time scrubbing for a case.

Palmer, L. (2013) Anaesthesia 101 – everything you need to know. *Plastic Surgical Nursing,* 33(4): 164–171.

If you want to learn more about anaesthesia, this is a really useful starting point. It goes over the drugs used and key considerations.

Trigo, A. (2016) 'Monitoring during anaesthesia and recovery.' *Nursing Management,* 23(8): 10.

This article provides an account of patient monitoring during anaesthesia and recovery which will help you when undertaking placements in theatre.

Annotated useful websites

World Health Organization. Safe Surgery Saves Lives. (2008). Available from: http://www.who.int/patientsafety/safesurgery/ss_checklist/en/index.htm

Using the WHO checklist: www.youtube.com/watch?v=CsNpfMldtyk

Useful resource of best evidence for healthcare practice – This particular page focuses on a specific area of perioperative practice: www.cochrane.org/search/site/surgical%20scrubbing

Twitter site which may be of use for those who feel they do not have time to check up on the latest findings: https://twitter.com/CochraneUK

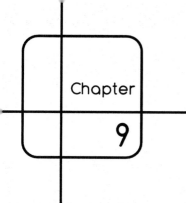

Chapter 9

Palliative care settings

Mike Bater and
Xiaodong Wu

(Continued)

6.4   understand the principles and processes involved in supporting people and families with a range of care needs to maintain optimal independence and avoid unnecessary interventions and disruptions to their lives.

Chapter aims

By the end of this chapter, you should be able to:

- acknowledge how multidisciplinary teams (MDTs) support end-of-life care patients in palliative care.
- identify transferable and specialist skills that can be learnt when undertaking symptom management during a palliative care placement.
- describe learning from undertaking a placement in supporting end-of-life patients in various settings.

Introduction

This chapter will identify the types of placement areas where you may be involved in end-of-life care as a Nursing Associate (NA) student. We will first explore how you may be feeling about such a placement, and how to prepare for it. The chapter will then consider some of the learning opportunities in these settings, and the key concepts in palliative care. These will be valuable for you in a range of other settings during your programme and as an NA student. There then follow three main sections outlining the learning you can expect to gain from a palliative care setting:

- working within the MDT towards a 'good death'
- symptom management and pain control
- physiological and psychological changes as death approaches

Where might a palliative care placement be?

As an NA student, you may experience palliative care in a range of settings such as a hospital ward (medical, surgical, elderly care, oncology), as it is shown that 50% of deaths occur in a hospital setting (Gold Standards Framework, 2017). You may also have an experience within a care home, Macmillan cancer team or in a hospice setting.

Preparing for placements in palliative care

It is useful to research your placement prior to starting, as discussed in Chapter 1. You will need to make contact in order to know the start date and times of your first shift and this can provide the opportunity to ask questions regarding the placement. This initial contact may be brief, but you may be able to obtain details on how to find more information.

On your first day of placement, you will have a comprehensive induction. This will include introducing you to the MDT, showing you around the placement, an explanation of the working environment and routine, as well as explaining the safety requirements.

Learning opportunities in a palliative care setting

When considering learning in palliative care settings it is useful to think about the transferable skills which you can take to other care settings. These skills include:

- *Communication*: You will encounter patients who are feeling sad, anxious or apathetic, who are crying and who may have altered communication patterns, social isolation and withdrawal. This can be seen as a learning opportunity to consider how you may adapt your communication skills to meet the needs of patients. In addition, you will experience how nurses speak to patients' loved ones either to deliver an update on the progress of the patient or to engage in significant discussion, and in some situations how they inform about a loved one's death over the phone.
- *Symptom management*: Pain and associated symptoms are essential parts of palliative care. A placement in a hospice provides an excellent opportunity to understand the biopsychosocial management of pain and associated symptoms such as nausea and vomiting, constipation and diarrhoea.
- *Pain management using a syringe driver*: There are several reasons why syringe pumps are used to give patients medicine:
  - The patients have nausea or vomiting.
  - They have difficulty swallowing oral medicine (for example, tablets).
  - Their symptoms cannot be managed well with oral medicine.
  - To avoid having to give injected medicines frequently.
  - They cannot absorb oral medicines effectively.
- *Psychological care*: Hospices manage patients' anxiety and depression with advanced cancer or other life-limiting diseases. This provides the opportunity for you to identify the individual patient's need, and the rationale for care.
- *Social aspects of care*: Grief is a normal reaction to bereavement or loss. It manifests differently in each individual (Royal College of Nursing, 2020).

This provides the opportunity for you to observe the bereavement process and those members of the MDT involved.

- *Spiritual aspects of care*: Palliative care is based on caring for the whole person, and what is important to them. This provides the opportunity to understand different religions' needs and practices.

The above points are not exhaustive and you will have different opportunities in some palliative care settings, such as wound care, mouth care, hygiene needs and pressure area care. You are encouraged to use your placement involving end-of-life care and caring for palliative patients to reflect on your learning and how you can utilise the experience in your future practice.

Working within the multidisciplinary team towards a 'good death'

NICE (2019, p. 6) states that 'End of life care is defined by NHS England as care that is provided in the "last year of life"; although for some conditions, end of life care may be provided for months or years'.

The aim of end-of-life care is primarily conservative, and aimed at giving comfort and maintaining quality of life, commonly referred to as palliative care. The aims of palliative care are to provide relief from pain and other distressing symptoms, integrate holistic care (physical, psychological, social and spiritual wellbeing) to enable people to live as actively as possible until their death (NICE, 2019).

Engaging with individuals, their family and the wider care team can provide learning opportunities to inform your future practice. Working with specialist practitioners in the support of individuals and families can inform your learning and expose you to positive role models. To benefit from what can feel like challenging or stressful situations you should take the opportunity to reflect on events to make sense of them and their outcomes.

Activity 9.1   Reflection

You have been allocated a placement that involves palliative and end-of-life care.

- What does palliative care and end-of-life care mean to you? This may include some 'myths' about palliative care.
- What feelings do you have in anticipation of undertaking the placement?

An outline answer is given at the end of the chapter.

Providing care of the dying person encompasses a wide range of skills that you can develop in this setting. These include pain and other symptom management and psychological, social, spiritual and bereavement support for their loved ones. A number of barriers have been identified to providing optimum end-of-life care, including the patient and their family members' avoidance of death, misleading posts on social media and lack of continuity and consistency of care. Ideally, quality care occurs when patients who are facing death and their loved ones are able to have honest, informed conversations in order to have the time to consider the meaning of their lives, and to make plans to prepare for a peaceful death.

Who is the multidisciplinary team in palliative care settings?

Palliative care is delivered through teamwork with a variety of healthcare professionals from the MDT. When you are on placement, you will have the opportunity to work with the MDT and this will add to a wider learning experience. This could in fact become one of your learning outcomes. Alongside working with other professionals, you will be welcomed to attend ward rounds and MDT meetings where the care of complex patients is comprehensively discussed. The MDT may include:

- doctor (consultant, registrar, junior doctor, medical student)
- nursing team (matron, ward manager, registered nurse, NA, student nurse, NA student)
- physiotherapist
- occupational therapist
- speech and language therapist (SaLT)
- dietitian
- social worker
- safeguarding team (adult and child)

During your placement, you should discuss with your practice assessor (PA) / practice supervisor (PS) to arrange a time when you can shadow some of the above MDT members; this will be a valuable learning experience for you.

Additionally, if undertaking a placement in a hospice, you will have the opportunity to learn about complex disease management and ethics related to decision making. Activity 9.2 asks you to engage with evidence-based practice in relation to advanced care planning.

Case study: Jane

Jane is 69 years old; she has dysphagia and was admitted to hospital due to a haemorrhagic stroke. Jane was referred to the SaLT for her swallowing difficulty. While in the hospital, Jane developed late-onset hospital-acquired pneumonia and was started on intravenous antibiotics. A further assessment indicated that Jane's condition had worsened and that she now appeared to lack capacity to express her

(Continued)

> (Continued)
>
> preferences for care. There was no formal advance statement about her future care needs. Jane's sister, who is next of kin, tells you that Jane did not wish to spend her last days in a hospital or hospice, but in her own home.
>
> A best-interest meeting is a multidisciplinary meeting that is arranged for a specific decision related to Jane's care.

Activity 9.2   Evidence-based practice

After reading the above case study about Jane, consider the following questions:

- What to expect at the meeting?
- Who will be there?
- Who makes the decision?
- What if the family member doesn't agree?

An outline answer is given at the end of the chapter.

The learning from Activity 9.2 can be applied in all end-of-life care settings, especially if patients have not completed the 'advanced care planning' process. The transition from active treatment to conservative care can be a stressful time for the individual, family and carers. Effective communication with the involvement of the individual and family in decision making can reduce the impact of these stresses. The Mental Capacity Act (2005) supports an individual to ensure their views are heard, or can be presented by an advocate in order to inform decision making. The implementation of advanced care planning following Jane's stroke would also provide representation of her wishes when later she lost capacity. This can occur during the treatment of her dysphagia prior to any implementation of palliative care. Preparing for the worst whilst hoping for the best is often the most helpful perspective to take for both the individual and their family.

Advanced care planning is the conversation between individuals, their families and carers and the MDT looking after them about their future wishes and priorities for care (Gold Standards Framework, 2017). Advanced care planning provides for greater autonomy, choice and control, enabling a sense of retaining control, self-determination and empowerment for the dying individual. It reduces unwanted or futile invasive interventions and hospital admissions, guiding those involved in care to provide appropriate levels of treatment. Enhanced proactive decision making reduces the later burden on the family and relieves anxiety in bereavement (Gold Standards Framework, 2017).

There are five steps within the Gold Standards Framework:

1. Think about the future; be clear as to what is important.
2. Talk with family and friends and ask someone to be spokesperson.

3. Record your thoughts and who is the nominated spokesperson.
4. Discuss your plans with the doctor and nurses to address any treatment issues.
5. Share this information with others who need to know.

Symptom management and pain control

In your programme, you will have learned about clinical skills such as monitoring the patient's vital signs: blood pressure, pulse, temperature, respiratory rate and oxygen saturations. This learning increases in complexity as you progress. For example, in Year 1 you would learn anatomy and physiology, and some pathophysiology. In Year 2, it is likely you will learn about how to apply such learning to increasingly complex clinical scenarios involving a range of treatments.

In palliative care, the biological changes at end of life determine the type and intensity of symptoms that individuals might experience. The changes that occur in organ failure are progressive and require monitoring and adjustment of interventions. The following section will look at some of the common distressing symptoms that may occur at the end of life, using a case study about Kwasi.

Case study: Kwasi

Kwasi is a 52-year-old man who is a heavy smoker and has end-stage chronic obstructive pulmonary disease (COPD) and stage 4 lung cancer with metastases. No further treatment is being offered to him. Kwasi has had another episode of deterioration; now he is bed-bound, has been unable to take food for more than a week and he is finding it difficult to drink water without considerable effort. You are the NA student looking after Kwasi.

- What are the signs and symptoms Kwasi might be experiencing?
- Do you think Kwasi is aware that he is approaching the end of his life?
- What would make you think this is the case? What are your priorities for his care?
- In which setting would you commonly see patients like Kwasi?

We will now discuss what informs the care needed in this case study.

It is often difficult to be certain that a person is dying, as each patient is different. It is essential to recognise the signs of dying in order to provide appropriate end-of-life care (National Palliative and End of Life Care Partnership, 2015). For Kwasi, the primary diagnosis is stage 4 lung cancer metastases; it has already spread to other organs, such as bone, lymph nodes and brain (Cancer Research UK, 2021). The underlying condition of COPD, caused by the lungs exchanging gases resulting in reduced oxygen saturation and hypoxia, could lead to breathlessness and anxiety. There are four stages to caring for Kwasi.

Stage 1: recognising the dying phase

It is likely that Kwasi is in the deteriorating or dying phase based on clinical evidence: disease trajectory and prognosis. Stage 4 lung metastases, reduced mobility, inability to take food, progressive weakness and fatigue indicate a significant biological change; the terminal phase may last hours to days.

Stage 2: communication with the patient, family and loved ones

This step involves communicating our understanding of the situation with family and loved ones. This is a vital step, as you may know that Kwasi is deteriorating, but the family and loved ones may be oblivious. The communication of the goals of his care is key to optimising comfort and dignity in order to prepare for the dying phase. Consider the setting you are in: if you are in the community or a care home, make sure anticipatory (just-in-case) medicine is available; if not, then inform the GP. If you are in the hospice, follow the local protocol; make sure that the next-of-kin contact details are up to date.

As an NA student undertaking a placement in a palliative care setting, you should try to remember the following acronym PREPARED (Clayton et al., 2007). This will help you communicate and care for a patient during end of life care.

- *P – prepare*: understand the medical condition and Kwasi's current status, considering the environment.
- *R – rapport*: show empathy and compassion.
- *E – expectations*: understand patient's and caregivers' expectations, considering cultural factors.
- *P – provide* information in simple, clear language and ensure a consistent approach.
- *A – acknowledge* their emotions and concerns.
- *R –* foster *realistic* hope.
- *E – encourage* questions and information; ask open questions to enable further discussion.
- *D – document* the discussion clearly on the nursing notes.

Stage 3: symptom management

In order to provide optimised comfort and dignity of care, the NA student needs to consider adequate symptom management and psychosocial and spiritual issues in order to balance the situation and facilitate a good death. Kwasi is likely experiencing physical symptoms – pain, dyspnoea, nausea and vomiting – and psychological symptoms that include anxiety, depression and confusion.

A syringe driver is the most appropriate device to use for managing complex symptoms. A syringe driver delivers continued subcutaneous infusion, as the oral route may not be feasible due to dysphagia, severe nausea and weakness. This is a common choice in the community setting as frequent subconscious injections are not practical (Watson et al., 2016).

Pain is a unique symptom and it is important to remember that not all cancer patients will have pain; according to Cancer Research UK (2021), around 65% of people with advanced cancer have pain. It is likely that Kwasi already had a pain management plan in place and this should be reviewed. The common practice is to constantly adjust the dosage of pain relief to optimise pain management and minimise side effects, such as nausea and vomiting and constipation. Due to the deterioration in his condition, the syringe driver is likely to be used; the syringe driver normally contains opioids; anti-emetics and anxiolytics. It may also include other medication such as anti-secretory drugs if necessary. The NA should assess pain regularly using appropriate tools, as Kwasi may be experiencing breakthrough pain, and this should include additional subcutaneous doses. Here is an example of the PQRST assessment tool (Swift, 2015):

- Palliative/provocative factors: what makes the pain worse?
- Quality: describe the pain.
- Radiation: where is the pain? (There may be pain at more than one site.)
- Severity: compare this pain to other pain previously experienced or the pain in the same location but at a previous time.
- Temporal factors/time: when did the pain start? How long does it last for? How often does the patient get the pain? What time of day is the pain better or worse?

(Swift, 2015)

Dyspnoea, also called breathlessness, is a very common symptom in COPD and advanced lung cancer patients. The NA student, along with the nurse, should assess what triggered dyspnoea, looking for reversible cues, as well as associated symptoms such as a productive cough and the colour of his sputum, and any source of infection, especially in the community setting. If any reversible cues are present, the NA student should inform the registered nurse / doctor/ GP to reassess the patient. Often dyspnoea can be triggered by strong emotions such as fear of dying, concern for loved ones or pets or spiritual concerns, which need to be acknowledged. Dyspnoea is often short-lived, and can be managed by both pharmacological and non-drug measures. Normally, it can be managed by prescribing benzodiazepines, such as sublingual lorazepam. Benzodiazepine medication can be beneficial to reduce anxiety, which compounds the perception of dyspnoea. If Kwasi is still very distressed or anxious due to persistence of the dyspnoea, then midazolam could be administered as part of anticipatory medication.

Stage 4: ethical decision making

If Kwasi's death is imminent, his family might ask for supporting interventions such as artificial hydration. It is important to remember that death is an irreversible pathological progress which occurs naturally and that artificial hydration does not prolong life (NICE, 2015). It is necessary to provide oral care, including frequent sips of fluid or ice cubes to promote comfort. It is important to make shared decisions on various issues such as rationalisation of medication; establishing Kwasi's wishes regarding preferred place of death; normally the patient has already stated this in their advanced care planning. The NA student role is to support patients and their family members as death becomes inevitable.

Sometimes, the patient knows that they are dying and can gradually have reduced cognitive function, or may become socially withdrawn. Some patients may develop restlessness, confusion and agitation. Physical signs include being peripherally cyanosed; they are cold to touch, normally starting from the extremities. Apnoea and altered breathing pattern are common, such as Cheyne–Stokes respiration – a pattern of respiration characterised by alternating periods of apnoea and deep, rapid breathing (NICE, 2015).

The above section discussed the 'deteriorating' and 'dying' phase of end-of-life care. The next section is focused on how to manage the 'stable' phase of palliative care. In this phase Kwasi is stable, symptoms are adequately controlled and his family / carer situation is relatively stable with no apparent new issues. As mentioned above, anticipatory medication will be prescribed if the patient is likely to die within a year (Table 9.1).

Table 9.1 Anticipatory medication, 'just in case' medication: examples (Johnstone, 2017)

Action	Medication	Indication
Analgesic	Morphine sulphate 10 mg/ml ampoules	Pain, breathlessness
Anti-emetic	Levomepromazine 25 mg/ml ampoules	Nausea and vomiting
Anxiolytic	Midazolam 10 mg/ml ampoules	Anxiety, distress
Anti-secretory	Hyoscine butyl bromide 20 mg/ml ampoules	Respiratory secretions

There are different types of pain medication for different types of pain, therefore the PQRST assessment, previously mentioned, or a simple scoring system which determines the severity of the pain, such as that of Wylde et al. (2011), can inform the pain management decision. International guidelines set out the types of pain medication that are most effective for different levels of pain; this is known as the analgesic ladder, and it recommends specific types of pain management for mild, moderate and severe pain (World Health Organization, 1986):

- mild pain – mild pain medication or anti-inflammatory drugs, for example, paracetamol
- moderate pain – weak opioid pain medication such as codeine
- severe pain – strong opioid pain medication, for example, morphine

Each step of the ladder is supported by other steps that can modify the pain, such as simple rest or elevation of a limb and the use of heat or cold to modify the sensation of pain. Additionally, other medications are often used to reduce spasm or anticonvulsant drugs are given for neuropathic pain (NICE, 2015).

The use of opioids or anxiolytic medication to reduce pain and anxiety can be effective in anxiety management and the suppression of a cough. These can be offered in discussion with the individual, their family and the MDT. Good symptom control in itself can reduce the impact of anxiety on breathing.

Nausea and vomiting are complex and may occur due to organ failure, the use of medications such as opioids, psychological causes or biochemical changes. The effects of pain, breathlessness and anxiety on Kwasi may have contributed to the psychological causes. When possible, the reversible causes of nausea and vomiting should be addressed, such as drug-induced, or chemical imbalance such as hypercalcaemia. Interventions such as reviewing the medication dose or the use of an alternative drug and correction of dehydration can reduce the effect of hypercalcaemia and resulting nausea and vomiting. The addition of an anti-emetic such as haloperidol to combat the effect of opioids can be effective and it is good practice that this is then reviewed daily. Although haloperidol is known as an antipsychotic medication, it can also be used as an anti-emetic when given at a low dose in palliative care (Murray-Brown and Dorman, 2015).

The above symptoms must not be viewed in isolation as they can exacerbate each other. Oral symptoms may also affect the individual's quality of life; such as dry lips, dry mouth, fungal and bacterial infections, coated tongue, gingivitis, ulcers and treatment-related side effects such as radiation stomatitis. These symptoms can result in local pain, anorexia or changes in appetite, and increased risk of respiratory infection.

The final section of this chapter will look at the physiological and psychological changes as death approaches using a case study on Christine.

Physiological and psychological changes as death approaches

As mentioned before, good palliative care is not just providing support to patients and their loved ones in the last month, days or hours, but also about enhancing the quality of life for patients at every stage of their diagnosis. Active disease management will decline and symptom management becomes the priority. This needs to be discussed by the MDT at every stage when the treatment plan is reviewed, especially when an intervention is changed or withdrawn. Good patient assessment, and pharmacological and non-pharmacological management are essential in controlling symptoms seen at the end of life. A holistic approach is essential as psychological symptoms such as depression can be under-recognised when managing physical symptoms such as pain. There is often a link between the meaning of pain and low mood experienced by individuals as they become more dependent on others for basic care (Marie Curie, 2020). Social isolation can exacerbate the experience of depression or low mood and simple screening questions on how the individual feels can initiate a discussion on mental wellbeing.

Earlier identification of people nearing the end of their life can be challenging for healthcare professionals in any setting. There is often uncertainty about how long a person has left to live and the signs that suggest someone is at the end of life can vary between individuals (Gold Standards Framework, 2017). General indicators of decline such as loss of mobility and anorexia are present alongside specific indicators relating to the location of the specific tumours or disease, such as having a metastatic stage 4 lung cancer and end-stage COPD.

In the end-of-life care setting, communication is not only sharing information, but it is also a tool for emotional support and care. Due to biological and psychological changes, communication can be difficult with patients and their loved ones. It is necessary to repeat the information several times so that they can absorb the information and feel reassured.

Four types of awareness are associated with patients who are dying:

1. *Closed awareness*: the patient does not recognise or denies that he or she is dying although everyone around knows.

2. *Suspected awareness*: the patient suspects what others know and attempts to confirm or negate it.
3. *Mutual pretence awareness*: everyone knows that the patient is dying but pretend to each other they do not know.
4. *Open awareness*: the patient, staff and relatives admit that death is inevitable and speak and act accordingly.

(Glaser and Strauss, 1965, cited in Andrews, 2015)

Advanced care planning (as discussed previously in relation to Jane) can prepare individuals, their family and the MDT to engage with decision making at the end of life.

Case study: Christine

Christine is a 91-year-old woman who lives in a care home and has end-stage heart failure, osteoarthritis and increasing signs of agitation. Following a fall, she has become less active, is eating less, is easily confused and has had repeated infections. Christine's daughter Stella has asked for the GP to review her mother's medication as she thinks it is contributing to her increasing frailty and agitation.

You are part of the MDT involved in Christine's care.

*   What are the physiological changes that are occurring?
*   What are the priorities of care that need to be discussed with Christine and her daughter Stella?
*   How should the team respond to a request from Stella to continue treatment of Christine's heart failure with drugs such as diuretics?
*   How should the team approach the discussion of withdrawing or withholding treatment?

We will now work through this case study.

There are a number of physiological changes for Christine. She has end-stage heart failure, which means the heart has a reduced ability to circulate oxygenated blood to the vital organs. She has breathlessness and a reduced response by the kidneys to treatment by diuretics, resulting in the formation of oedema. She has a poor appetite, which is often associated with gastrointestinal oedema or the development of ascites, both of which can reduce stomach capacity. Disruption in diet can result in constipation, which is often exacerbated by analgesic medications containing codeine. Fatigue associated with heart failure and reduced mobility increases towards the end of life. A dry mouth is often associated with reduced food and fluid intake, which is normal at the end of life due to fluid shifting out of the vascular compartment and into the tissues as oedema. Co-morbidities such as osteoarthritis can become more painful with reduced activity and require changes to the type or dose of medication. Agitation is a term that describes anxious, restless and unsettled behaviour linked to emotional, physical or spiritual distress.

The review of Christine provides the opportunity for the MDT to help Stella to recognise the possibility that Christine is dying. Answering Stella's questions about her mother's symptoms and the changes in treatment required can facilitate shared decision making and identify personal needs for Christine at the end of life. The involvement of Stella can help with the sense of helplessness families feel when watching others provide care for their relative at the end of life.

Withholding or withdrawing treatment might be viewed as 'giving up' by relatives who are not involved in the discussion of treatment. The inclusion of Christine in decision making can facilitate the discussion of her end-of-life wishes with Stella and the MDT.

With focus of care being the promotion of comfort, the MDT and Stella can plan for death, such as using sedation for agitation or strong pain relief, instituting a 'do not attempt resuscitation' status for Christine and the meeting of her spiritual needs.

The involvement of carers and family in the end-of-life process can support them in the initial days of bereavement and provide a resource for the follow-up of the bereaved.

Chapter summary

This chapter began by providing examples of how to prepare for clinical placements with a particular focus on palliative care settings. The specialist skills discussed originate from good holistic care and can be transferred into non-palliative care situations to inform your practice. Learning from the palliative care setting will help you identify common symptoms and the need for effective communication with the MDT. The application of holistic care to complex symptom management has identified the need for good team working within the MDT to meet the needs of the individual.

Activities: brief outline answers

Activity 9.1 Reflection

- What is palliative care?

Palliative care is treatment, care and support for people with a life-limiting illness, and their family and friends. It is sometimes called 'supportive care' (Marie Curie, 2020).

Myth: Having palliative care means you are going to die soon.
Fact: Some people receive palliative care for years, while others will receive care in their last weeks or days.
Myth: Palliative care means you no longer receive active treatment.
Fact: Palliative care continues alongside treatments such as chemotherapy and radiotherapy.

- What is end-of-life care?

End-of-life care involves treatment, care and support for people who are nearing the end of their life. It is an important part of palliative care (Marie Curie, 2020).

End-of-life care normally refers to people who are expected to die within 6–12 months, and is an important part of palliative care (Marie Curie, 2020). In 2004, the World Health Organization stated that palliative care should integrate care for people with any condition who may die in the foreseeable future (Murray et al., 2017). Three trajectories are summarised below:

1. Trajectory 1: rapid decline (cancer); this is predictable decline in physical health over a period of months or years. Patients probably have reduced function and are unable to maintain self-care.
2. Trajectory 2: intermittent decline (organ failure), in a condition like end-stage chronic obstructive pulmonary disease, heart failure or end-stage renal failure. Patients likely have ongoing illness for years; deteriorations are generally associated with hospitalisation and intensive treatment. It is difficult to predict death, as each episode of exacerbation may result in death.
3. Trajectory 3: gradual decline (physically frail and dementia); progressive cognitive and physical impairment could be caused by an acute event such as a fall, fracture or pneumonia.

- What feelings do you have in anticipation of undertaking the placement?

Like any new encounter, we are faced with unknown reactions from others and ourselves. You may feel anxious about talking to individuals who are aware that they are dying; you may be worried about saying something wrong. You may have had previous experiences that evoke strong feelings such as sadness. It is important to recognise your feelings and discuss them with your practice supervisor or practice assessor so that support can be offered.

Activity 9.2 Evidence-based practice

- What to expect at the meeting?

The meeting will be an open forum for all interested parties to provide the relevant information with regard to specific decisions that need to be made relating to the patient's care/treatment. This meeting will enable a fully informed decision to be made about a particular aspect of the person's care or treatment.

- Who will be there?

Attending the meeting will be allied healthcare professionals relevant to the specific decision, e.g doctor, nurse, SaLT, dietitian, physiotherapist, occupational therapist and adult social care worker. It is good practice to involve the family in order for them to advocate on the known wishes of the patient.

- Who makes the decision?

If the decision is in relation to health (e.g. long-term feeding), the consultant will be the decision maker unless there is an appointed lasting power of attorney for health and welfare, including life-sustaining treatment.

- What if the family member doesn't agree?

If next of kin are not in agreement with the final decision, there is a right to approach the Court of Protection regarding complex decisions.

Annotated further reading

NICE (2019) NICE Guideline 142. *End of Life Care for Adults: Service Delivery.* Available at: www.nice.org.uk/guidance/ng142 (accessed 19 March 2021).

This guideline covers organising and delivering end-of-life care services, which provide care and support in the final weeks and months of life (or, for some conditions, years), and the planning and preparation for this. It aims to ensure that people have access to the care that they want and need in all care settings. It also includes advice on services for carers.

NICE (2011) *End of Life Care for Adults.* Available at: www.nice.org.uk/guidance/qs13/resources/end-of-life-care-for-adults-pdf-2098483631557 (accessed 8 July 2021).

This quality standard covers care for adults (aged 18 and over) who are approaching the end of their life. This includes people who are likely to die within 12 months, people with advanced, progressive, incurable conditions and people with life-threatening acute conditions.

NICE (2019) *End of Life Care for Infants, Children and Young People with Life-limiting Conditions: Planning and Management.* Available at: www.nice.org.uk/guidance/ng61 (accessed 8 July 2021).

This guideline covers the planning and management of end-of-life and palliative care for infants, children and young people (aged 0–17 years) with life-limiting conditions.

NICE (2015) NICE Guideline ng31. *Care of Dying Adults in the Last Days of Life.* Available at: www.nice.org.uk/guidance/ng31 (accessed 19 March 2021).

This guideline covers the clinical care of adults (18 years and over) who are dying during the last 2–3 days of life. It aims to improve end-of-life care for people in their last days of life by communicating respectfully and involving them, and the people important to them, in decisions and by maintaining their comfort and dignity.

Smith, R. (2000) A good death: an important aim for health services and for us all. *BMJ*, 320: 129. Available at: www.bmj.com/content/bmj/320/7228/129.full. pdf?casa_token=2lg8v5WHEA4AAAAA:Na0jhmn-T_UHtiwexLUjRn8sPjkdloAv 9VkBhigcZRiR07Wu8dDOUkkzODYurht-CFW81S8jx0o (accessed 26 February 2021).

This article revisits the attitudes of healthcare professionals towards discussing death with individuals and the need to discuss dying as part of holistic care.

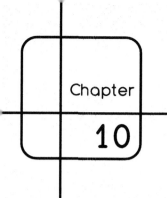

Chapter 10

Child and young people care settings

Sophie McKay

Chapter aims

After reading this chapter, you should be able to:

- demonstrate awareness of the different placement areas within child and young people (CYP) settings.
- identify the stages of communication development in children and gain skills in delivering developmentally appropriate communication techniques while undertaking a placement within CYP settings.
- describe the importance of early years and childhood experiences and the potential impacts this can have on life choices and in later life.
- identify the principles of adolescent assessment including the HEEADSSS assessment tool (*home* environment, *education*, *eating* habits, *activities* and peer relationships, *drug* and alcohol use, *sexuality*, *suicidal* thoughts and depression and *safety*) and explore the common communication barriers with adolescents.
- demonstrate awareness of immunisation and vaccination applicable to the CYP setting.
- demonstrate understanding of nutrition and hydration and explore how to calculate fluid allowance for infants, children and young people.

Introduction

This chapter will explore the variety of experiences you can gain from undertaking a placement within the CYP care setting. The stages of paediatric communication development will be explored and there will be tips on how to engage with children and young people. Early years and childhood development will be discussed, and this chapter will explore how abuse in the early years can negatively affect later childhood and adult life. This chapter will introduce the HEEADSSS (*home* environment, *education*, *eating* habits, *activities* and peer relationships, *drug* and alcohol use, *sexuality*, *suicidal* thoughts and depression and *safety*) assessment tool and how to apply this when interacting with adolescents and young people (Cohen et al., 1991). You can learn a wide range of skills within the CYP settings, and many of those skills are transferable to other care settings. This chapter will also include communication, nutrition and hydration, health screening tools, immunisation and vaccination in relation to CYP.

Student tip 10.1

Child placements vary so much and can be quite specialised. It is important to get as much information as you can about your placement so you can prepare. It could be in a GP setting, so it would be great to read up on immunisation, or it could be in Child and Adolescent Mental Health Services (CAMHS), so it would be great to read up on HEEADSSS!

Toni, Year 1 Nursing Associate (NA) student

CYP settings have a number of specialist areas that you may have the opportunity to experience during your training. Before you start a CYP placement, it is important for you to know some of these common areas. The most common areas are listed below, so you can familiarise yourself with the diverse environments where a CYP may be cared for whilst they are unwell or receiving treatment:

- general paediatric ward
- health visitor (based in either a community clinic or patient's house)
- community nursing
- school nursing
- paediatric intensive care unit (PICU)
- neonatal intensive care unit (NICU)
- paediatric emergency department
- paediatric outpatients
- children's hospice
- children's short stay units
- CAMHS
- Tier 4 acute general adolescent mental health units (specialist inpatient CAMHS unit)
- specialist paediatric wards, such as: cardiac, haematology, oncology, surgical, orthopaedic, respiratory, trauma or specialist eating disorder or CAMHS mental health unit

Communication in child and young people settings

The six Cs were published by NHS England in 2016 as a *Compassion in Practice* initiative to provide a set of values for all healthcare staff (NHS England, 2016). When caring for patients across healthcare settings we must strive to do so in line with the six Cs, listed below:

- communication
- courage
- care
- compassion
- commitment
- competence

(NHS England, 2016)

Learning how to communicate with children and young people is therefore an important learning outcome when undertaking a placement within CYP settings. Communication is described as a fundamental skill of nursing and we must strive to communicate clearly with patients of all ages (Denieul and Robinson, 2019). Effective communication will support healthcare staff with gaining patient consent and support and providing updates for the patient and family. It is important that all communication between the nurse and patient is clear, transparent, honest and respectful.

To deliver effective communication to a CYP it is important to understand their developmental age. This will enable efficient communication whereby the CYP can understand and make sense of the situation or task that is being asked of them. Quite often children respond well to healthcare practitioners who display warm, trusting, engaging and developmentally appropriate verbal language (Price and McAlinden, 2018). In order to gain as much as you can from your CYP placement you will need to take all these factors into consideration. Interacting with children in pain, or fearful children, will enhance your communication skills. You can then apply these transferable communication skills to other areas of nursing, such as mental health and learning disabilities.

Stages of communication development in children

Children generally go through three phases of communication development, which are intentional, symbolic and linguistic communication (Brown and Elder, 2014). Crying is a pre-verbal form of social interaction; the newborn infant will use this communication technique to signal for attention and help from others so their nutritional and care needs can be met. In the first year of life infants develop a basic understanding of all their senses: sight, smell, taste, touch and hearing.

Intentional communication

Intentional communication can be described as communicating through basic vocalisation or use of body language with intent to signal for a particular need (Price and McAlinden, 2018). This can be witnessed in the final months of infancy when infants begin to motion either vocally or physically to express their needs or desires. An example of this is crying or a particular vocalisation that is consistently associated with a specific request, such as hunger. The infant has created basic communication by signalling vocally for a particular need and the parent or carer is able to understand that this individualised vocalisation is associated with the infant being hungry. As an NA student you should respond to a crying infant in a timely way, making sure your tone of voice is calming and soothing. When soothing a baby, you should consider what the baby is trying to signal for. For example, are they hungry, in pain, uncomfortable in a wet nappy, uncomfortable and needing to be burped, or are they anxious because they are alone and want to be held? Thinking about what the baby is signalling for will help you identify how to soothe the baby and meet their needs. When caring for a baby over a few days you may start learning that baby's specific intentional communication, and you may be able to identify their individualised vocalisation to signal for a particular need.

Symbolic communication

Symbolic communication can be described as using primary language in its most basic form to communicate with others (Price and McAlinden, 2018). This is typically observed in toddlers and young children and is characterised by them using short sentences or words to describe their needs. They may use this communication to interact with others, gain attention and for social development. The toddler age group (1–3 years) are often fearful of strangers and this should be considered when building a rapport with them. You should take time to observe the toddler's interaction with their parents and then engage with both the parents and child; if the parent accepts this communication the toddler will likely do so as well. Children in this age group often use simplified words for objects. A good way to engage with the toddler is to learn these words and use them when communicating with them so the language is one that they understand. Such as, 'Do you need to use the toilet?' versus 'Do you need to peepee'? The toddler may be familiar with the term 'peepee' and unfamiliar with the word 'toilet' so considering this you will be able to communicate with them according to their developmental age. A key learning opportunity is therefore learning to care for the toddler, in close partnership with the parents.

Siblings are also a great asset when communicating with this age group. An older sibling might try to help you communicate with their sibling by giving you tips such as, 'She only eats her breakfast with her orange spoon', or 'My sister might swallow the medication if you sing her favourite song to her'. A toddler might also be comforted and more likely to engage with you if you are positively engaging with their siblings and parents.

Children aged 3–5 years are highly creative; they love to explore and play, so often the best way to communicate and build a rapport with this age group is through play. Engaging through play can decrease stress and anxiety, provide a distraction from unpleasant procedures and help the child make sense of a new experience. Further reading on this is suggested at the end of the chapter. Please note when communicating with this age group that simplified words and sentences should be used as they do not yet understand a complex vocabulary.

Activity 10.1   Critical thinking

During your placement, you are asked by your practice supervisor (PS) to escort a 3-year-old patient to have an ultrasound scan of their abdomen. Using the above information on communication and developmental stages, how might you introduce yourself to the patient and their parents? How would you prepare the patient for this scan?

An outline answer is given at the end of the chapter.

Linguistic communication

Linguistic communication is developed in late childhood or adolescence and can be described as the most sophisticated phase of communication development (Price and McAlinden, 2018). When a person uses linguistic communication, they can use all types of communication to engage with another person. The young person who has met their communication and developmental milestones will be able to make sense of the information you are sharing with them. It is important to consider that the young person is not fully emotionally mature and will still require the same support and care given to a younger patient, just delivered in a developmentally appropriate way.

The HEEADSSS assessment

The HEEADSSS assessment is a tool or prompt which was introduced to aid healthcare professionals in identifying and establishing the psychosocial needs of an adolescent or young person (Cohen et al., 1991). Awareness of this tool will enable you to understand the complex issues that can affect the physical and emotional wellbeing of adolescents and young people. The HEEADSSS assessment includes the following:

- *H*: home situation, family life, relationships and stability
- *E*: education/employment
- *E*: eating and exercise
- *A*: activities and peer relationships
- *D*: drug use, cigarettes and alcohol
- *S*: sexuality, gender identity and safe sexual practices
- *S*: suicide, self-harm, depression and coping strategies
- *S*: safety, risk-taking behaviours and environment

The HEEADSSS assessment is used to assess the adolescent's activities of daily living and to examine areas they might need help with (Cohen et al., 1991). While undertaking a CYP placement you will have the opportunity to learn about and undertake a HEEADSSS assessment. The needs and challenges of adolescent patients can be unique and different to the needs of a child or adult; many healthcare workers find the HEEADSSS tool extremely useful in identifying the needs of an adolescent. It is especially useful when approaching difficult topics such as drug use and safe sexual practices.

Student tip 10.2

I attended a child and adolescent placement in Year 1 and used the HEEADSSS assessment, which I found really interesting. Then in Year 2 I had a placement in an adult admission unit, and I brought my learning about HEEADSSS in when we had an angry young man as a patient; he was 18, so technically an adult, but in many ways presented younger than this. The HEEADSSS was a useful tool, and the staff there learned about it from me!

Andrew, Year 2 NA student

Importance of early years and infant mental wellbeing

In the 1930s, infant mental wellbeing was first explored by Sigmund Freud, who started by examining how the experiences of a child may affect them later in life and in adulthood. The negative experiences that children can be exposed to in their early years can affect their adulthood in many ways, such as motivation, resilience, emotional intelligence and mental health (Price and McAlinden, 2018). In some cases, these negative experiences can lead to destructive or risky behaviours, use of recreational drugs and violent tendencies and even leave the young adult susceptible to trafficking, modern slavery or sexual abuse. It is thought that early intervention in negative experiences brings about better outcomes later in life, thus it is vital that the CYP healthcare practitioner is alert and responds quickly to potential wellbeing threats to a child of any age.

A cross-party manifesto published by the NSPCC (NSPCC, Wave Trust and Pip UK, 2013) is used in the UK to identify the importance of the child's first 1001 days. Whilst on a CYP placement it is important that you familiarise yourself with the 1001 critical days publication as summarised in Table 10.1, as this will help you recognise and respond to wellbeing threats.

Table 10.1 The 1001 critical days (adapted from NSPCC, Wave Trust and Pip UK, 2013). See the full manifesto at: www.nspcc.org.uk/globalassets/documents/news/critical-days-manifesto.pdf

Key area	Description
Importance of the early years	This section draws attention to the United Nations human rights of a child and how all of these should be met in their early years. All children have the right to have a happy, healthy and supportive childhood free from abuse and harm
Parents and families at the heart of services	Ensures the support, guidance and education of parents to enable them to provide all needs for their children. If further parental support is required, this needs to be delivered in a timely manner and it needs to meet the needs of the child. Recognising fathers as positive role models and parenting equals is also within this section
Child development and early intervention	'The healthy child programme' is from pregnancy to age 5 and should be consistently and fully abided by
Skilled professionals	Professionals caring for children need to be trained and possess the skills to recognise and respond to wellbeing concerns
A strong relationship with the sector	Community children's services aim to provide targeted services that meet the individual needs of children in that community. Community healthcare practitioners should also have the knowledge required to signpost parents and children to relevant support services

The five sections of the 1001 critical days strategy outline the aspects key to preventing poor infant wellbeing. These strategies are put in place to safeguard infants' physical, mental and emotional wellbeing so they have the best chance to grow and develop into their full potential (Price and McAlinden, 2018).

Health screening in children and young people

During your CYP placement, you may be asked to assist in health screening of infants and children. We will now explore the current health screening service provided in the

UK for children and young people. Health screening promotes the early identification of illness and diseases to enable early treatment and prevention of disease progression. The *Healthy Child Programme* (Department of Health, 2009) is a national incentive to promote the wellbeing, health and development of all children from birth to 19 years of age (Denieul and Robinson, 2019). Community practitioners such as health visitors, midwives, school nurses and community nurses deliver this programme. This national programme aims to assess the child's development and progress and to give health and wellbeing advice to the child and family. The areas of advice may include child growth and development, healthy eating and infant nutrition, maternal mental health, child and adolescent mental health, bullying and sexual health.

The UK health screening for CYP includes:

- antenatal screening
- assessment of maternal mental health
- newborn baby examination
- newborn hearing screening before 4 weeks of age
- baby review at 2 weeks old
- visual and hearing tests at 4–5 years old
- health needs assessment at 10–12 years old
- national child measurement in height and weight in reception class and Year 6

(Denieul and Robinson, 2019).

A newborn screening blood test is taken at 5 days old; this is often referred to as the Guthrie test, named after Robert Guthrie, an American physician who developed it in 1962. This blood test is taken via a heelprick test and screens for certain recessive genetic disorders, including cystic fibrosis, maple syrup urine disease, phenylketonuria, sickle-cell disease, hyperthyroidism/hypothyroidism, congenital adrenal hyperplasia, galactosaemia and other specific genetic and metabolic syndromes. If the test returns positive for any of these conditions the parents are informed. An early diagnosis can lead to efficient planning and care for the child. This heelprick test is usually carried out by CYP nursing staff either in the community or in a hospital setting. Undertaking the heelprick test requires skill and attention to detail, and this is something you are likely to assist with whilst on placement. More information on heelprick tests can be found at: www.nhs.uk/conditions/baby/newborn-screening/blood-spot-test/

Development reviews are included in the health screening of the CYP. These reviews take place at 6–8 weeks, 9–12 months and 2 years to assess how the child is growing and developing. They aim to assess each part of the child's development – hearing and sight, physical, emotional and cognitive development – to ensure the child is meeting their developmental milestones. Whilst on your CYP placement you will observe these development reviews. It is important that you understand the milestone markers and can recognise the normal development of CYP and identify if they are not meeting these milestones so you can escalate this and get the child further support.

Under-5-year-olds' medical history, such as immunisation record, height, weight and head circumference, is recorded in an A5 red book given to the family shortly after the baby is born. Each child is different and reaches their development milestones at different times. It is therefore useful for CYP healthcare practitioners to have some knowledge of the normal development and milestone characteristics so they can recognise signs of delayed development. For example, the seven main reflexes of the newborn should be present in a healthy infant. A delay in developing the seven main reflexes, particularly in the first few months of an infant's life, may be a sign of developmental delay and as such further investigations would be required.

Seven main reflexes of the newborn

Developmental checks are part of health screening in CYP settings. When caring for an infant it is important that you can recognise the seven main reflexes of a newborn. In developmentally healthy newborns these seven reflexes will be present and if they are absent in this age group you should escalate this to your PS. If these reflexes are present in an older child, this can be a sign of developmental delay and should also be escalated and documented appropriately.

1. *Rooting* – the infant turns their cheek in response to touch, searching for something to suck, such as the mother's breast.
2. *Sucking* – when the roof of the baby's mouth is touched, they will begin to suck. This reflex is developed at gestational week 32, thus some premature infants may find it difficult to carry out the sucking reflex.
3. *Swallowing* – this reflex works in conjunction with the sucking reflex and allows the infant to draw the milk into the oesophagus and to the stomach.
4. *Moro* – if the infant is startled, they will arch their back and throw their arms open.
5. *Grasp* – if you introduce your finger to a baby's hand, they will curl their fingers and grasp yours.
6. *Babinski* – the baby's toes will spread and curl inwards when the sole of their foot is stroked.
7. *Stepping* – the baby will imitate walking movements when held in an upright position with their feet touching a surface.

(Davies and McDougall, 2019)

Immunisation and vaccination in child and young people's nursing

The saying 'an ounce of prevention is worth a pound of cure', attributed to Benjamin Franklin in the 1700s, is still relevant today to describe the importance of ill-health prevention as it can avoid needing to cure or treat a disease in later life. Learning about immunisation and vaccination will help you provide evidence-based information to families when they are considering vaccinating their children. Immunisation is arguably the most successful public health intervention and can bring about decreased incidences of preventable infectious diseases. Due to the smallpox vaccine, smallpox was declared globally eradicated in 1980. However, in recent years we have seen an upward trend in childhood vaccine-preventable infectious diseases here in the UK. Within an inpatient CYP setting you may have the opportunity to care for patients with pertussis (whooping cough), measles, mumps or meningococcal group B, even though these diseases are preventable through childhood vaccinations. In the UK, many childhood vaccinations are free and because of this it is quite rare for children to become unwell with measles or mumps. This may have led some parents to become more concerned regarding the risks associated with the vaccine rather than their child becoming unwell with the infectious disease. In 1988, a research article was published that supposedly linked the MMR vaccine to the development of autism; this led some parents to reject and refuse this vaccine. Although this research article has since been discredited, sadly this myth can still be heard today as a reason for vaccine refusal.

All healthcare practitioners delivering immunisations should understand both the benefits and the potential side effects in order to deliver evidence-based information to parents so an informed decision can be made. Table 10.2 outlines the immunisation programme for children in the UK; familiarity with this schedule will help you while you are undertaking a placement in CYP settings.

Table 10.2 Immunisation programme for children in the UK (Public Health England, 2020)

Age due	Diseases protected against	Vaccine given and trade name		Usual site
8 weeks old	Diphtheria, tetanus, pertussis (whooping cough), polio, *Haemophilus influenzae* type B (Hib) and hepatitis B (HepB)	DTaP/IPV/Hib/HepB	Infanrix hexa	Thigh
	Meningococcal group B	MenB	Bexsero	Left thigh
	Rotavirus	Rotavirus	Rotarix	By mouth
12 weeks old	Diphtheria, tetanus, pertussis, polio, Hib and HepB	DTaP/IPV/Hib/HepB	Infanrix hexa	Thigh
	Pneumococcal (13 serotypes)	Pneumococcal conjugate vaccine (PCV)	Prevenar 13	Thigh
	Rotavirus	Rotavirus	Rotarix	By mouth
16 weeks old	Diphtheria, tetanus, pertussis, polio, Hib and HepB	DTaP/IPV/Hib/HepB	Infanrix hexa	Thigh
	MenB	MenB	Bexsero	Left Thigh

Age due	Diseases protected against	Vaccine given and trade name		Usual site
1 year old (on or after the child's first birthday)	Hib and MenC	Hib/ MenC	Menitorix	Upper arm/ thigh
	Pneumococcal	PCV booster	Prevenar 13	Upper arm/ thigh
	Measles, mumps and rubella	MMR	MMR VaxPRO or Priorix	Upper arm/ thigh
	MenB	MenB booster		Left thigh
Eligible paediatric age groups	Influenza (each year from September)	Live attenuated influenza vaccine (LAIV)	Fluenz Tetra	Both nostrils
3 years 4 months old or soon after	Diphtheria, tetanus, pertussis and polio	dTaP/IPV	Repevax or Boostrix-IPV	Upper arm
	Measles, mumps and rubella	MMR (check first dose given)	MMR VaxPRO or Priorax	Upper arm
Boys and girls aged 12–13 years	Cancers caused by human papillomavirus (HPV) types 16 and 18 (and genital warts caused by types 6 and 11)	HPV (two doses given 6–24 months apart)	Gardasil	Upper arm
14 years old (school Year 9)	Tetanus, diphtheria and polio	Td/IPV (check MMR status)	Revaxis	Upper arm
	Meningococcal groups A, C, W and Y disease	MenACWY	Nimenrix or Menveo	Upper arm

During your CYP placement, you will have the opportunity to observe the childhood immunisation programme. You can observe important clinical skills such as injection technique, medication preparation and administration. When observing clinical skills such as injection technique you must always abide by the NMC Code of Conduct (2018d) and work within your limits of practice.

Nutrition, hydration and elimination

You may be assigned by your PS to assist with the nutritional care of the child. This may include assisting with feeding of children of all ages and documenting volumes and totals clearly. Therefore, it is important you have some understanding of this in preparation for your placement. Children will grow and develop when they receive adequate nutrition with a balanced intake of macro- and micronutrients to meet their basic metabolic needs. Macronutrients include proteins, carbohydrates and lipids. Micronutrients include minerals such as iron, copper, zinc, vitamins, phosphate, calcium and magnesium. An infant with adequate nutrition can be expected to double their birth weight by 6 months of age and quadruple it by the time they are 2 years old. A child's metabolic rate reaches the maximum rate at age 2, then decreases with age. Good nutrition in childhood is vital for wellbeing, growth and development.

Infants are usually breastfed or formula-fed, or a combination of both. The UNICEF breastfeeding initiative (UNICEF, 2013) evaluates research studies that outline the benefits of breastfeeding. Benefits include lower rates of inpatient admissions with gastroenteritis and respiratory conditions of the newborn. Due to maternal health, breast milk supply and prematurity some infants are not able to breastfeed. Mothers should be fully supported in their personal choice of feeding method. To support the breastfeeding mother, you will need to make the environment comfortable and ensure she is adequately fed and hydrated.

Current UK advice suggests infants should start weaning from exclusive milk feeds to some solid foods around 6 months old. Infants and children should always be supervised when eating due to the risk of choking; in particular small round foods such as grapes should always be cut in half to reduce this risk. Some infants are ready before or after 6 months to start weaning and the type of weaning foods varies. It can be spoon-feeding puréed food or soft finger food.

In infants around 80% of their body weight is water, and clinical dehydration can occur when an infant loses more than 5% of that water. Dehydration can occur in infants due to intolerance of feeds, viruses or diarrhoea and vomiting. Common signs of dehydration in the infant can be tachycardia, lethargy, irritability, reduced skin turgor, sunken eyes and appearing unwell.

Children usually begin toilet training between 2 and 3 years. Before this age, children will use their nappies when eliminating waste. In order to catch a urine sample for an infant you will need to clean the nappy area, cover the bedsheets with an absorbent pad and wait vigilantly to catch the urine – you may want to ask the parents to help you with this. In the toddler age group, you can place a specimen pot into a clean potty to collect the urine.

Case study: Victor

Victor has been allocated a placement on a CYP ward. Although Victor has gained a lot of experience on adult placement areas, this placement will be Victor's first in a CYP area. Victor contacts the placement area before starting and discusses with his allocated PS if there is anything he needs to do to prepare for this placement. Victor's PS emails him activities and reading for him to complete; that will help him prepare for his CYP placement. Activity 10.2 outlines one of the activities sent to Victor.

Activity 10.2 Critical thinking

In Table 10.3 you will find the common formulas used to calculate daily fluid allowances for CYP patients. Using the formula and scenarios given, calculate the fluid allowance for each child. This will help you familiarise yourself with these calculations in preparation for your CYP placement.

Table 10.3 Daily fluid allowance calculations

Formula	Scenario	Answer
100 ml/kg for the first 10 kg 50 ml/kg for the second 10 kg 20 ml/kg for each subsequent kg (This will give you the total fluid allowance for 24 hours; to get the hourly rate divide your answer by 24)	Evie weighs 24 kg and has been prescribed intravenous fluids. Work out the hourly rate for her fluids Connor weighs 41 kg and has been prescribed intravenous fluids. Work out the hourly rate for his fluids	
120 ml/kg/day 120 × weight Divide by 24 to get the hourly rate, then multiply by the frequency	Naya weighs 4.7 kg and is being fed every 2 hours with expressed breast milk. What 2-hourly volume would you give? Emily weighs 3.9 kg and is being fed every 3 hours with formula milk. What 3-hourly volume would you give?	

An outline answer is given at the end of the chapter.

Chapter summary

This chapter has explored the stages of child development and strategies to support developmentally appropriate communication for CYP patients. Early years and childhood development were explored alongside a detailed discussion on how infant wellbeing and developmental stages can affect a child in later life. The HEEADSSS assessment was introduced and an explanation given of how to apply it when interacting with adolescents. The chapter ended with a brief overview of health screening and immunisation for children and young people.

Activities: brief outline answers

Activity 10.1 Critical thinking

During this activity you may want to consider how you would introduce yourself to the patient, how you might alter your body language and the words you use. You may also wish to involve a play specialist or see if the child's parents can come in for this intervention.

If the parent is present, start by engaging with them in a warm and friendly manner, then introduce yourself to the 3-year-old. You could start the interaction by asking, 'What's your name?', 'How old are you?' Then move on to a toy or teddy they have brought with them and ask what the teddy's name is. Compliment the teddy as this will help the toddler warm to you. Next you need to prepare the patient for the ultrasound scan. Due to the patient's developmental age you need to do so with short sentences and words and incorporate play in your explanation. You could do so in the following way: 'The doctor needs to take a picture of your tummy, I'll show you on teddy'. Then speak to teddy and ask. 'Are you ready for your special tummy picture?' Animate teddy, saying 'Yes', then show the toddler through play that to get the picture the doctor will use a funny wiggly pen with slippery gel on it to slide it on teddy's tummy, then it will show a picture on the screen. Tell the toddler that teddy was very good because he stayed very still and the doctor took a great picture. Then explain, 'Now teddy has had his picture it is your turn'. Then it would be good to accompany the patient during the scan so you can narrate the procedure just as you did when you were describing it through play.

Activity 10.2 Critical thinking

The answers, and how to work them out, are shown in Table 10.4.

Table 10.4 Daily fluid allowance calculations: answers

Formula	Scenario	Answer
100 ml/kg for the first 10 kg 50 ml/kg for the second 10 kg 20 ml/kg for each subsequent kg (This will give you the total fluid allowance for 24 hours; to get the hourly rate divide your answer by 24)	Evie weighs 24 kg and has been prescribed intravenous fluids. Work out the hourly rate for her fluids	100 ml × 10 kg = 1000 ml 50 ml × 10 kg = 500 ml 20 ml × 4 kg = 80 ml 1000 + 500 + 80 = 1580 ml (total fluid allowance in 24 hours) 1580 ÷ 24 (to get the hourly rate) = 65 ml/hour
	Connor weighs 41 kg and has been prescribed intravenous fluids. Work out the hourly rate for his fluids	100 ml × 10 kg = 1000 ml 50 ml × 10 kg = 500 ml 20 ml × 21 kg = 420 ml 1000 + 500 + 420 = 1920 ml (total fluid allowance in 24 hours) 1920 ÷ 24 (to get the hourly rate) = 80 ml/hour

Formula	Scenario	Answer
120 ml/kg/day 120 × weight Divide by 24 to get the hourly rate, then multiply by the frequency	Naya weighs 4.7 kg and is being fed every 2 hours with expressed breast milk. What 2-hourly volume would you give?	120 × 4.7 = 564 ml (total fluid allowance in 24 hours) 564 ÷ 24 (to get the hourly rate) = 23.5 23.5 × 2 (to get the volume to be fed every 2 hours) = 47 ml
	Emily weighs 3.9 kg and is being fed every 3 hours with formula milk. What 3-hourly volume would you give?	120 × 3.9 = 468 ml (total fluid allowance in 24 hours) 468 ÷ 24 (to get the hourly rate) = 19.5 19.5 × 3 (to get the volume to be fed every 3 hours) = 58.5 ml

Annotated further reading

app.heeadsss.uk

This app provide guidance for completing the HEEADSSS assessment.

Barry, P., Morris, K. and Ali, T. (2017) *Paediatric Intensive Care*. Oxford: Oxford University Press.

This book has lots of useful information if your placement is in a paediatric intensive care unit (PICU).

Davies, J.H. and McDougall, M. (2019) *Children in Intensive Care*, 3rd ed. London: Elsevier.

This book has lots of useful information if your placement is in a paediatric intensive care unit (PICU).

Macqueen, S., Bruce, E. and Gibson, F. (2012) *The Great Ormond Street Hospital Manual of Children's Nursing Practices*. Chichester, West Sussex: Wiley-Blackwell.

This is a really useful book that gives a step-by-step guide on how to deliver clinical interventions to the child or young person.

References

Alzheimer's Society (2021) *A Specialist Hospital Ward for People with Dementia.* Available at: www.alzheimers.org.uk/dementia-together-magazine/feb-march-2017/specialist-hospital-ward-people-dementia (accessed: 3 February 2021).

Amstein, A. (1969) A ladder of participation. *Journal of the American Institute of Planners,* 35(4): 216–224.

Andrews, T. (2015) Awareness of dying remains relevant after fifty years. *Grounded Theory Review,* 14.

Asthma UK (2019) *The Great Asthma Divide.* Available at: www.asthma.org.uk/58a0ecb9/globalassets/campaigns/publications/The-Great-Asthma-Divide.pdf (accessed 15 February 2021).

Bowen, J. (2017) How to get the most out of your placement in the emergency department. *BMJ,* 359. doi: https://doi.org/10.1136/sbmj.i4429.

Brown, A.B. and Elder, J.H. (2014) Communication in autism spectrum disorder: a guide for pediatric nurses. *Pediatric Nursing,* 40(5): 219–225. Available at: https://pubmed.ncbi.nlm.nih.gov/25929112/ (accessed 28 February 2021).

Cancer Research UK (2021) *Lung Cancer: Stages, Types and Grades.* Available at: www.cancerresearchuk.org/about-cancer/lung-cancer/stages-types-grades/stage-4 (accessed 26 February 2021).

Clayton, J., Hancock, K., Butow, P., Tattersall, M. and Currow, D. (2007) Clinical practice guidelines for communicating prognosis and end-of-life issues with adults in the advanced stages of a life-limiting illness, and their caregivers. *MJA,* 186: S77–S108.

Cohen, E., MacKenzie, R.G. and Yates, G.L. (1991) HEADSS, a psychosocial risk assessment instrument: implications for designing effective intervention programs for runaway youth. *Journal of Adolescent Health,* 12(7): 539–544.

CQC (2020) *The State of Care.* Available at: www.cqc.org.uk/publications/major-report/soc201920_0b_summary (accessed 9 February 2021).

Davies, J.H. and McDougall, M. (2019) *Children in Intensive Care,* 3rd ed. London: Elsevier.

Day-Calder, M. (2017) Get the most out of your practice placements. *Nursing Standard,* 31(19): 35.

Dementia Statistics (2021) *Prevalence by Age in the UK.* Available at: www.dementiastatistics.org/statistics/prevalence-by-age-in-the-uk/ (accessed 16 June 2021).

Dementia UK (2021) What is Dementia? Available at: www.dementiauk.org/get-support/diagnosis-and-next-steps/what-is-dementia/ (accessed 3 February 2021).

Denieul, V. and Robinson, J. (2019) *Children's Nursing Placements*. London: Lantern Publishing.

Department of Health (2001) *Valuing People: A New Strategy for Learning Disability for the 21st Century*. London: Department of Health.

Department of Health (2005) *Mental Capacity Act*. London: HMSO.

Department of Health (2009) *Healthy Child Programme: Pregnancy and the First Five Years of Life*. Available at: https://assets.publishing.service.gov.uk/government/uploads/system/uploads/attachment_data/file/167998/Health_Child_Programme.pdf (accessed 16 June 2021).

Department of Health (2013) *Information: To Share or not to Share. The Government's Response to the Caldicott Review (2013)*. Available at: https://assets.publishing.service.gov.uk/government/uploads/system/uploads/attachment_data/file/251750/9731-2901141-TSO-Caldicott-Government_Response_ACCESSIBLE.PDF (accessed 8 July 2021).

DoHSC (2021) *Integration and Innovation: Working Together to Improve Health and Social Care for All*. Available at: https://assets.publishing.service.gov.uk/government/uploads/system/uploads/attachment_data/file/960548/integration-and-innovation-working-together-to-improve-health-and-social-care-for-all-web-version.pdf (Accessed 12 February 2021).

Dougherty, L. and West-Oram, A. (2015) The Royal Marsden Manual of Clinical Nursing Procedures. New York: John Wiley.

Driscoll, J. (1994) Reflective practice for practise. *Senior Nurse*, 14(1): 47–50.

Dutton, H. and Finch, J. (2018) *Acute and Critical Care Nursing at a Glance*. Oxford: Wiley Blackwell.

Equality Act (2010) c. 15. Available at: www.legislation.gov.uk/ukpga/2010/15/contents (accessed 28 February 2021).

Flaherty, C. and Taylor, M. (2021) *Developing Academic Skills for Nursing Associates*. London: Learning Matters.

General Data Protection Regulation (2018) *Data Protection Act*. London. HMSO. Available at: www.legislation.gov.uk/ukpga/2018/12/contents/enacted (accessed 26 February 2021).

Glaser, B.G. and Strauss, A.L. (1965) *Awareness of Dying*. Chicago, IL: Aldine Publishing.

Gold Standards Framework (2017) *Advance Care Planning in 5 Simple Steps*. Available at: www.goldstandardsframework.org.uk/advance-care-planning (accessed: 26 February 2021).

Government (1990) *The National Health Service and Community Care Act*. London: HMSO.

Grady, P.A. and Gough, L.L. (2014) Self-management: a comprehensive approach to management of chronic conditions. *American Journal of Public Health*, 104(8): e25–e31.

Hatfield, A. and Tronson, M. (2009) *The Complete Recovery Room*. Oxford: Oxford University Press.

References

Heslop, P., Blair, P., Fleming, P., Hoghton, M., Marriott, A. and Russ, L. (2013) *Confidential Inquiry into Premature Deaths of People with Learning Disabilities.* Bristol: Norah Fry Centre for Disability Studies. Available at: www.bristol.ac.uk/media-library/sites/cipold/migrated/documents/fullfinalreport.pdf (accessed 8 July 2021).

HM Government (2018) *Working Together to Safeguard Children: A Guide to Inter-agency Working to Safeguard and Promote the Welfare of Children.* Available at: https://assets.publishing.service.gov.uk/government/uploads/system/uploads/attachment_data/file/942454/Working_together_to_safeguard_children_inter_agency_guidance.pdf (accessed 16 June 2021).

Jaul, E., Barron, J., Rosenzweig, J.P. and Menczel, J. (2018) An overview of co-morbidities and the development of pressure ulcers among older adults. *BMC Geriatrics*, 18. Available at: https://link.springer.com/article/10.1186/s12877-018-0997-7 (accessed 15 February 2021).

Johnstone, L. (2017) Facilitating anticipatory prescribing in end-of-life care. *The Pharmaceutical Journal.* Available at: https://pharmaceutical-journal.com/article/ld/facilitating-anticipatory-prescribing-in-end-of-life-care#main-content (accessed 9 April 2021).

Kings Fund (2018) *Making Sense of Integrated Care Systems.* Available at: www.kingsfund.org.uk/publications/making-sense-integrated-care-systems#developing (accessed 1 February 2021).

Knaak, S., Mantler, E. and Szeto, A. (2017) Mental illness-related stigma in healthcare: barriers to access and care and evidence-based solutions. *Healthcare Management Forum*, 30(2): 111–116.

Kottner, J., Cuddigan, J., Carville, K., Balzer, K., Berlowitz, D., Law, S., Litchford, M., Mitchell, P., Moore, Z., Pittman, J., Sigaudo-Roussel, D., Yee Yee, C. and Haesler, E. (2019) Prevention and treatment of pressure ulcers/injuries: the protocol for the second update of the International Clinical Practice Guideline 2019. *Journal of Tissue Viability*, 28: 51–58.

Marie Curie (2020) *What are Palliative Care and End of Life Care?* Available at: www.mariecurie.org.uk/help/support/diagnosed/recent-diagnosis/palliative-care-end-of-life-care (accessed 26 February 2021).

Mayo Clinic (2020) *Dementia.* Available at: www.mayoclinicF.org/diseases-conditions/dementia/symptoms-causes/syc-20352013 (accessed 12 February 2021).

McGee, E.M. (2006) The healing circle: resiliency in nurses. *Issues in Mental Health Nursing*, 27: 43–57.

Mehigan, S. (2021) Reflective writing. In: Flaherty, C. and Taylor, M. (eds.) *Developing Academic Skills for Nursing Associates.* London: Learning Matters, pp. 75–86.

Mental Capacity Act (2005) *Code of Practice.* Available at: https://assets.publishing.service.gov.uk/government/uploads/system/uploads/attachment_data/file/921428/Mental-capacity-act-code-of-practice.pdf (accessed: 26 February 2021).

Mental Health Act (1983) c. 20 Available at: www.legislation.gov.uk/ukpga/1983/20/section/136 (accessed 16 June 2021).

Miller, W.R. and Rollnick, S. (2013) *Motivational Interviewing: Helping People Change*, 3rd ed. New York: Guilford Press.

Montague, J., Crosswaite, K., Lamming, L., Cracknell, A., Lovatt, A. and Mohammed, M.A. (2019) Sustaining the commitment to patient safety huddles: insights from eight acute hospital ward teams. *British Journal of Nursing*, 28(20). Available at: www.magonlinelibrary.com/doi/full/10.12968/bjon.2019.28.20.1316 (accessed 1 February 2021).

Murray, S.A., Kendall, M., Mitchell, G., Moine, S., Amblàs-Novellas, J., Boyd, K. et al. (2017) Palliative care from diagnosis to death. *BMJ*, 356: j878. Doi:10.1136/bmj.J878.

Murray-Brown, F. and Dorman, S. (2015) Haloperidol for the treatment of nausea and vomiting in palliative care patients. *Cochrane Database of Systematic Reviews*. Available at: www.ncbi.nlm.nih.gov/pmc/articles/PMC6481565/pdf/CD006271.pdf (accessed 12 May 2021).

National Palliative and End of Life Care Partnership (2015) *Ambitions for Palliative and End of Life Care*. Available at: http://endoflifecareambitions.org.uk/wp-content/uploads/2015/09/Ambitions-for-Palliative-and-End-of-Life-Care.pdf (accessed 26 February 2021).

NHS (2019a) *NHS Health Check*. Available at: www.nhs.uk/conditions/nhs-health-check/ (accessed 25 February 2021).

NHS (2019b) *Overview: Peripheral neuropathy*. Available at: www.nhs.uk/conditions/peripheral-neuropathy (accessed 9 July 2021).

NHS (2020) *About Dementia: Dementia Guide*. Available at: www.nhs.uk/conditions/dementia/about/ (accessed 10 February 2021).

NHS Digital (2020) *Health and Care of People with Learning Disabilities*. Available at: https://digital.nhs.uk/data-and-information/publications/statistical/health-and-care-of-people-with-learning-disabilities (accessed 4 March 2021).

NHS Employers (2019) *Employer Guide to Nursing Associates*. Available at: www.nhsemployers.org/nursingassociates (accessed 16 June 2021).

NHS England (2014) *Five Year Forward View*. Available at: www.england.nhs.uk/wp-content/uploads/2014/10/5yfv-web.pdf (accessed 13 February 2021).

NHS England (2016) *Compassion in Practice*. Available at www.england.nhs.uk/wp-content/uploads/2016/05/cip-yr-3.pdf (accessed 8 March 2021).

NHS England (2017) *Next Steps on the Five Year Forward View*. Available at: www.england.nhs.uk/wp-content/uploads/2017/03/NEXT-STEPS-ON-THE-NHS-FIVE-YEAR-FORWARD-VIEW.pdf (accessed 12 February 2021).

NHS England (2019) *The Long-Term Plan*. Available at: www.longtermplan.nhs.uk/ (accessed 12 February 2021).

NICE (2011) *Common Mental Health Problems: Identification and Pathways to Care*. Available at: www.nice.org.uk/guidance/cg123/resources/common-mental-health-problems-identification-and-pathways-to-care-pdf-35109448223173 (accessed 16 June 2021).

References

NICE (2015) NICE Guideline ng31. *Care of Dying Adults in the Last Days of Life.* Available at: www.nice.org.uk/guidance/ng31 (accessed 19 March 2021).

NICE (2018a) Alcohol – Problem Drinking: *Scenario: Alcohol Misuse.* Available at: https://cks.nice.org.uk/topics/alcohol-problem-drinking/management/alcohol-misuse/ (accessed 16 June 2021).

NICE (2018b) *Anaemia – iron deficiency.* Available at: https://cks.nice.org.uk/topics/anaemia-iron-deficiency/ (accessed 22 April 2021).

NICE (2019) NICE Guideline 142. *End of Life Care for Adults: Service Delivery.* Available at: www.nice.org.uk/guidance/ng142 (accessed 19 March 2021).

NMC (2018a) *Standards of Proficiency for Registered Nursing Associates.* Available at: www.nmc.org.uk/standards/standards-for-nursing-associates/standards-of-Proficiency-for-nursing-associates/ (accessed 16 June 2021).

NMC (2018b) *Standards for Pre-registration NA Programmes.* London: NMC.

NMC (2018c) *Standards for Student Supervision and Assessment.* Available at: www.nmc.org.uk/globalassets/sitedocuments/standards-of-proficiency/standards-for-student-supervision-and-assessment/student-supervision-assessment.pdf (accessed 16 June 2021).

NMC (2018d) *The Code.* Available at: www.nmc.org.uk/standards/code/ (accessed 12 February 2021).

NSPCC, Wave Trust and Pip UK (2013) *The 1001 Critical Days: The Importance of the Conception to Age 2 Period.* Available at: www.nspcc.org.uk/globalassets/documents/news/critical-days-manifesto.pdf (accessed 8 March 2021).

OED (2021) 'social, adj. and n.' *OED Online*, Oxford University Press, December 2020, www.oed.com/view/Entry/183739 (accessed 9 February 2021).

Paton, F., Chambers, D., Wilson, P., Eastwood, A., Craig, D. Fox, D., Jayne, D. and McGinnes, E. (2014) Effectiveness and implementation of enhanced recovery after surgery programmes: a rapid evidence synthesis. *BMJ Open*, 4. Available at: www.google.co.uk/url?sa=t&rct=j&q=&esrc=s&source=web&cd=&cad=rja&uact=8&ved=2ahUKEwi2nvLfg4HvAhWooFwKHRlVDrsQFjAaegQIBhAD&url=https%3A%2F%2Fbmjopen.bmj.com%2Fcontent%2F4%2F7%2Fe005015&usg=AOvVaw1jKq6hjlZXvEjw12gQvGzy (accessed 23 February 2021).

Payne, R.A. (2016) The epidemiology of polypharmacy. *Clinical Medicine*, 16(5): 465–469.

Peate, I. (2019) *Learning to Care. The Nursing Associate.* London: Elsevier.

PHE (2020) *Guidance on the 5 Alcohol Use Screening Tests.* Available at: www.gov.uk/government/publications/alcohol-use-screening-tests/guidance-on-the-5-alcohol-use-screening-tests (accessed 16 June 2021).

PLPLG (2019) *The Pan London Practice Assessment Document. Nursing Associates.* Available at: https://plplg.uk/nursing-associates/ (accessed 16 June 2021).

Price, B. (2019) Improving nursing students' experience of clinical placements. *Nursing Standard*, 34(9): 43–49.

Price, J. and McAlinden, O. (2018) *Essentials of Nursing Children and Young People.* London: SAGE.

Public Health England (2015) NHS Health Check Competency Framework. Pdf.

Public Health England (2018) *Reasonable Adjustments for People with Learning Disabilities*. Available at: www.gov.uk/government/collections/reasonable-adjustments-for-people-with-a-learning-disability (accessed 28 February 2021).

Public Health England (2020) *The Complete Routine Immunisation Schedule from June 2020*. Available at: https://assets.publishing.service.gov.uk/government/uploads/system/uploads/attachment_data/file/849184/PHE_complete_immunisation_schedule_Jan2020.pdf (accessed 8 March 2021).

RCN (2021) *Clinical Governance*. Available at: www.rcn.org.uk/clinical-topics/clinical-governance (accessed 11 February 2021).

Resuscitation Council UK (2015) *The ABCDE Approach*. Available at: www.resus.org.uk/library/2015-resuscitation-guidelines/abcde-approach (accessed 16 December 2020).

Rowe, G., Counihan, C., Eillis, S., Gee, D., Graham, K., Henderson, M., Barnes, J. and Carter-Bennett, J. (2020) *The Handbook for Nurse Associates and Assistant Practitioners*, 2nd ed. London: SAGE.

Royal College of Nursing (2020) *End of Life Care / Bereavement*. Available at: www.rcn.org.uk/clinical-topics/end-of-life-care/bereavement (accessed 26 February 2021).

SCIE (2015) *Good Practice in Social Care with Refugees and Asylum Seekers*. Available at: www.scie.org.uk/publications/guides/guide37-good-practice-in-social-care-with-refugees-and-asylum-seekers/glossary.asp (accessed 2 March 2021).

Servellen, V. and Marram, G. (2020) *Communication Skills for the Health Care Professional: Context, Concepts, Practice and Evidence*. Burlington, VT: Jones and Bartlett Learning.

Shirey, M. (2009) Transferable skills and entrepreneurial strategy. *Clinical Nurse Specialist*, 23(3): 128–130.

Simper, T.N., Breckon, J.D. and Kilner, K. (2017) Effectiveness of training final-year undergraduate nutritionists in motivational interviewing. *Practice Education and Counseling*, 100: 1898–1902.

Skills for Care (2020) *The Size and Structure of the Adult Social Care Sector and Workforce in England*. Available at: www.skillsforcare.org.uk/adult-social-care-workforce-data/Workforce-intelligence/documents/Size-of-the-adult-social-care-sector/Size-and-Structure-2020.pdf (accessed 12 February 2021).

Smith, P., McKeon, A., Blunt, I. and Edwards, N. (2014) *NHS Hospitals under Pressure: Trends in Acute Activity up to 2022*. Available at: www.nuffieldtrust.org.uk/files/2017-01/hospitals-under-pressure-web-final.pdf (accessed 23 February 2021).

Sudore, R.L., Lum, H.D., You, J.J, Hanson, L.C. Meier, D.E., Pantilat, S.Z., Matlock, D.D., Rietjens, J.A.C., Korfage, I.J., Ritchie, C.S., Kutner, J.S., Teno, J.M., Thomas, J., McMahan, R.D. and Heyland, D.K. (2017) Defining advance care planning for adults: a consensus definition from a multidisciplinary Delphi panel. *Journal of Pain and Symptom Management*, 53(5): 821–832.e1. doi.org/10.1016/j.jpainsymman.2016.12.331

Swift, A. (2015) Pain management 3: the assessment of pain in adults. *Nursing Times*, 111(41): 12–17.

UK Government (2011) *No Health Without Mental Health: A Cross-Government Mental Health Outcomes Strategy for People of All Ages*. London: Department of Health. Available at: https://assets.publishing.service.gov.uk/government/uploads/system/uploads/attachment_data/file/138253/dh_124058.pdf (accessed 16 June 2021).

UNICEF (2013) *The Evidence and Rationale for the UNICEF UK Baby Friendly Initiative Standards*. Available at: www.unicef.org.uk/wpcontent/uploads/sites/2/2013/09/baby_friendly_evidence_rationale.pdf (accessed 8 March 2021).

Wanko Keutchafo, E.L., Kerr, J. and Jarvis, M.A. (2020) Evidence of nonverbal communication between nurses and older adults: a scoping review. *BMC Nursing*, 19: 53. doi.org/10.1186/s12912-020-00443-9

Watson, M., Armstrong, P., Black, I., Gannon, C. and Sykes, N. (2016) *Palliative Adult Guidelines*, 4th ed. Bedfordshire and Hertfordshire: London Cancer Alliance, Northern Ireland, PallE8, RM Partners, Surrey, Sussex and Wales.

World Health Organization (1986) *Cancer Pain Relief*. Geneva: Office of Publications, World Health Organization.

World Health Organization (2008) *Why Safe Surgery is Important*. Available at: https://www.who.int/teams/integrated-health-services/patient-safety/research/safe-surgery (accessed 8 July 2021).

Wylde, V., Hewlett, S., Learmonth, I. and Dieppe, P. (2011) Persistent pain after joint replacement: prevalence, sensory qualities, and postoperative determinants. *Pain*, 152(3): 566–572.

Index

Locators in **bold** refer to tables and those in *italics* to figures.